Easy Home Massage

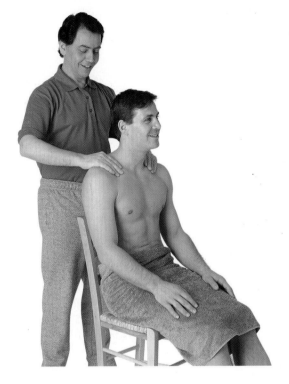

Mario Paul Cassar, D.O.

TIME
LIFE
BOOKS

Alexandria, Virginia

Time-Life Books is a division of Time Life Inc.

TIME LIFE INC.

PRESIDENT AND CEO: George Artandi

TIME-LIFE CUSTOM PUBLISHING

Vice President and Publisher — Terry Newell
Vice President of Sales and Marketing — Neil Levin
Director of Acquisitions and
Editorial Resources — Jennifer Pearce
Director of Creative Services — Laura McNeill
Director of Special Markets — Liz Ziehl
Project Manager — Jennie Halfant

First printing. Printed in China

TIME-LIFE is a trademark of Time Warner Inc. U.S.A.

Library of Congress Cataloging-in-Publication Data

Cassar, Mario Paul.
    Easy home massage / Mario Paul Cassar.
      p. cm. -- (Time-Life health factfiles)
    Includes index.
      ISBN 0-7370-1613-2 (pbk. : alk. paper)
      1. Massage. 2. Relaxation. I. Title. II. Series.
    RA780.5.C369 1999
    615.8'22--dc21   99-26882
                                              CIP

Books produced by Time-Life Custom Publishing are available at a
special bulk discount for promotional and premium use. Custom
adaptations can also be created to meet your specific marketing
goals. Call 1-800-323-5255.

A Marshall Edition
Conceived, edited, and designed by
Marshall Editions Ltd
The Orangery
161 New Bond Street
London W1Y 9PA

I dedicate this book to all my
family, especially my mother
Mary. Also to Zoë, Emma
and Laurie.

Note

Every effort has been taken to
ensure that all information in
this book is correct and
compatible with national
standards generally accepted at
the time of publication. The
author and publisher disclaim
any liability, loss, injury or
damage incurred as a
consequence, directly or
indirectly, of the use and
application of the contents of
this book.

CONTENTS

The Arms

Head and Shoulders

Self Massage

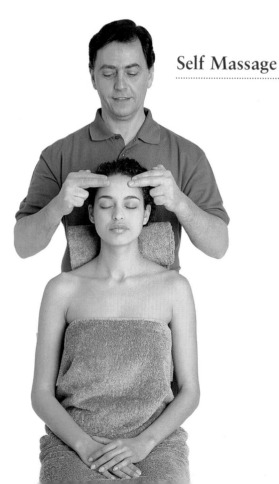

INTRODUCTION

Massage has been used throughout history, both for relaxation and as a means of applying healing ointments and oils to the skin. Although widely practised today, massage is still considered by some people as an exclusive luxury. This belief, however, is unjustified. It requires little effort, and no previous experience or special skills, to give a basic, relaxing massage. It is even possible to do an effective self-massage.

The guidelines presented in this book illustrate how to give a simple massage to someone lying on a massage couch. A couch is a useful, but not essential, accessory – you may find it easier to carry out the massage on the floor, or on any comfortable surface that is at the right height. And in certain situations, such as pregnancy, massage is more comfortable if the person being massaged sits on a chair or stool.

RELAXATION

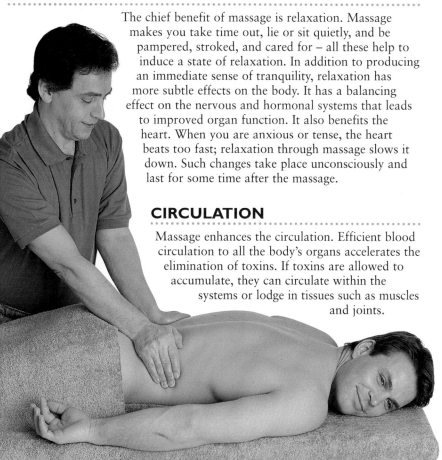

The chief benefit of massage is relaxation. Massage makes you take time out, lie or sit quietly, and be pampered, stroked, and cared for – all these help to induce a state of relaxation. In addition to producing an immediate sense of tranquility, relaxation has more subtle effects on the body. It has a balancing effect on the nervous and hormonal systems that leads to improved organ function. It also benefits the heart. When you are anxious or tense, the heart beats too fast; relaxation through massage slows it down. Such changes take place unconsciously and last for some time after the massage.

CIRCULATION

Massage enhances the circulation. Efficient blood circulation to all the body's organs accelerates the elimination of toxins. If toxins are allowed to accumulate, they can circulate within the systems or lodge in tissues such as muscles and joints.

Massage is also beneficial to the immune system. By stimulating kidney and bowel function, massage can aid the process of elimination. And massage increases the number of endorphins circulating in the blood; these are natural painkillers produced by the brain.

BENEFITS FOR MUSCLES

Muscles, especially those associated with posture, are frequently tense, most commonly because of incorrect posture and overuse of associated muscle groups. Stress, such as that caused by anxiety, has a similar effect. The relaxation induced by massage helps to ease muscle tension, especially tension associated with stress. Massage also loosens and stretches the muscles, and improves the blood supply to them.

A by-product of some massage strokes is heat. Increasing the temperature of body tissues helps to break up fatty deposits, and improved circulation helps to disperse them. This can slow down the formation of cellulite.

PRECAUTIONS

Massage is safe for most people. However, there are occasions when it is inadvisable. It is best not to massage someone who feels unwell, whether that is due to a simple cold or more complicated conditions such as migraine or inflammation. Pain and tenderness are useful indicators of body malfunction or injury, and it is wise to avoid massage in these circumstances.

Similar precautions apply to stomach aches, ulcers, skin infections, open wounds, broken bones, or unexplained heat and pain radiating down the leg or along the arm. An exception is the ache which follows prolonged use of a muscle. Tired, aching muscles are common after sports such as tennis, running, or bicycling. The discomfort is invariably due to an accumulation of metabolites (the by-products of metabolism) within the muscles, and in these cases it is safe to massage the area. If the pain is associated with a severe strain or tear, however, do not massage. Anyone with a serious condition, such as cancer or heart problems, or inflammatory arthritic conditions such as rheumatoid arthritis, should only be massaged by a professional massage therapist.

The commonsense approach to massage is to avoid it if there is any doubt about its safety.

MASSAGE ROUTINES

There are no rules as to where on the body a massage should begin or end. Examples of massage routines are given throughout the book, starting with massage to the back. This gives a beginner the opportunity to learn the massage movements on a relatively safe region of the body, and one that benefits most from massage. Working on this area is very rewarding and gives confidence to a person attempting his or her first massage. However, any of the routines can be reversed or changed about to suit both.

It is not essential to include the whole body, particularly if time is limited. A short massage concentrating only on the back, face, or feet is still relaxing.

MASSAGE STROKES

In this book massage movements are described as light for relaxation, medium for circulation, and deep for muscle tension. These are the dominant effects of the stroke but naturally there is an overlap between all the movements.
■ Light stroking is carried out with little pressure other than the weight of the hands; it can be compared to stroking a pet.
■ Medium pressure is a more positive movement with some added pressure.
■ Deep pressure massage is carried out only on muscles. It helps to loosen and stretch knotted muscle fibers.

LENGTH OF MASSAGE

The length of a massage can vary to suit the needs of the person being massaged and can take as long as one hour or as little as five minutes. A massage stroke is usually carried out three to five times but can be repeated as many times as necessary.

MASSAGING POSTURES

If you are going to give a massage, it is vital that you are comfortable and do not put any strain on your body. Any tension in the body or the hands of the masseur is easily transferred to the person being massaged.

All the routines in this book are demonstrated with you standing to give a massage and the person you are massaging lying on a massage couch. This is perhaps the most comfortable and convenient arrangement. However you can also carry out the routines on the floor, using a suitable padding. If you prefer to massage on the floor, you may find it most comfortable sitting with your legs crossed or with your legs straight, or kneeling.

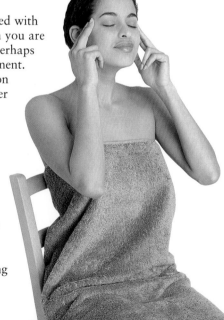

PREPARING FOR A MASSAGE

Massage and discomfort do not go together. Give yourself enough time to set up the space where the massage is to take place, and gather everything you need together so you do not interrupt the continuity of the massage. Low lighting and soft music are essential for creating a relaxing massaging atmosphere.

The body temperature tends to drop when a person lies down for a while, so increase the room temperature slightly: try turning up the thermostat half an hour or so before you begin the massage. In addition, cover the body of the person you are massaging with a blanket or towel, uncovering only the area you are working on.

CLOTHING

For comfort and freedom of movement, wear loose clothing with short sleeves when giving a massage. Both participants should remove shoes, belts, watches, rings and necklaces. As massage is ideally carried out on bare skin, the person being massaged should also remove some clothing, but how much you take off is a matter of personal preference.

MASSAGE OILS

Massage is best carried out using a massage oil or cream. These act as lubricants, allowing the hands to slide over the body surface without any friction. Use only a small amount, since too much oil or cream can cause the hands accidentally to slip off the body surface.

In addition to lubricating, some oils and creams introduce essences of herbs and flowers into the skin. Most drugstores, beauty shops, and health-food stores carry a selection of ready-mixed massage oils or creams. Alternatively, you can make your own by buying one of the essential oils used in aromatherapy and adding a few drops into a base oil such as wheat germ or sunflower. The most common essential oil, and invariably the most relaxing, is lavender. This is a safe, general purpose oil that can also be used on children. Camomile is also pleasant and safe.

Beyond these two oils the choice becomes a matter of preference. It is advisable, however, to ask for help when buying ready-mixed oils. While most are pleasant to use, some are intended for more specific purposes than relaxation. A few may have some side effects, and one or two may not be suitable at all. This is particularly important if you are going to be massaging a child or a woman who is pregnant or breastfeeding: always seek advice in these circumstances.

Talcum powder is not recommended. Although it is smooth and soothing, it clogs the pores.

SELF MASSAGE

The last chapter in this book describes a number of massage movements that are easy to use on yourself. When you massage yourself, you can vary the pressure and speed of the strokes as you wish. Self massage is also easy to do anywhere and at any time you find convenient.

The Back

I

THE BACK

The relaxing power of massage is perhaps more readily felt on the back than anywhere else in the body. This is partly because the effects of emotional tension are generally concentrated within the muscles of the upper back and shoulders. The back muscles also play a major role in supporting the posture, and are subjected to physical influences that cause them to become contracted and fatigued. The massage routines on the following pages begin with light strokes for relaxation, progressing to deeper massage to improve circulation and relieve tension. You can give a simple relaxing massage using only the light stroking movements. These strokes can also be applied to warm up the tissues and prepare the muscles for the deeper massage techniques.

STARTING BACK MASSAGE

Massage to the back starts with light-pressure strokes that are used primarily to relax the muscles and to prepare them for the deeper massage strokes. Light stroking is also a gentle way of establishing contact with the person you are massaging.

PREPARING A PERSON FOR MASSAGE

The same positions can be adopted for all the back massage sequences, unless otherwise specified for individual movements.

■ The person you are massaging should lie face down, with his head turned to whichever side is more comfortable.

■ Place a flat cushion or folded towel under the person's abdomen to prevent unnecessary hollowing of the back. Support his feet with a cushion or rolled-up towel, inserted under the ankle and the lower end of the shin bone. For extra comfort and support, place a soft pillow or cushion under the chest.

■ Cover the person's legs with a towel to prevent them feeling from cold during the massage.

WHERE TO STAND

Stand on whichever side of the massage couch is more convenient. Turn your body slightly so you are facing toward the person being massaged. Avoid excessive twisting of the back. Keep your weight evenly distributed on both legs.

Detail

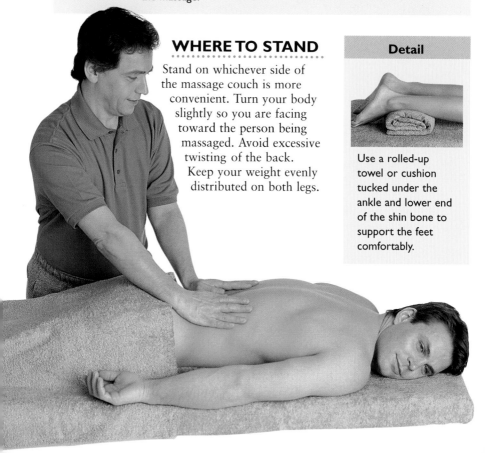

Use a rolled-up towel or cushion tucked under the ankle and lower end of the shin bone to support the feet comfortably.

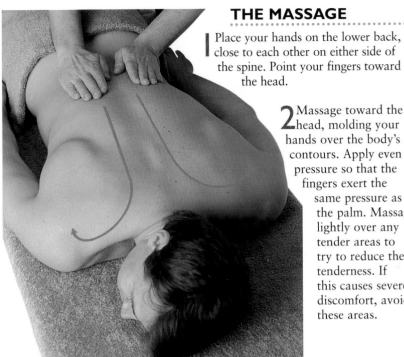

THE MASSAGE

1 Place your hands on the lower back, close to each other on either side of the spine. Point your fingers toward the head.

2 Massage toward the head, molding your hands over the body's contours. Apply even pressure so that the fingers exert the same pressure as the palm. Massage lightly over any tender areas to try to reduce the tenderness. If this causes severe discomfort, avoid these areas.

3 Continue the same light massage as you move to the upper back, working out to the shoulders. Cup each hand as you massage over the shoulders.

4 Flatten the hands and gradually massage down the outside of the trunk, as far as the pelvis, then take the hands back to the center of the lower back. Repeat a whole movement several times. Massage at a steady speed, the slower the better. Allow about 6 seconds to complete each movement.

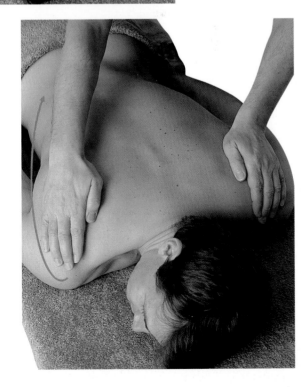

ACROSS THE BACK: *Light Stroke*

This light-pressure massage, carried out across the muscle fibers, helps to induce relaxation. Use it in addition to the light movement along the back (pp. 10–11) or as an alternative stroke. This movement can also be continued over the pelvis. Massage gently over any tender areas and avoid them completely if they are very sensitive.

WHERE TO STAND

Stand with your body facing across the massage couch. From this position you can comfortably reach the middle and lower back as well as the pelvis. Place one hand on the far side of the lower back. Set the other hand on the side nearest to you. Point the fingers of both hands away from you. Make contact with your whole hand – the heel, palm, and fingers.

Warming up

Massage is like any other form of exercise in that it is important to "warm up" gently before starting a more vigorous routine. Always carry out these light massage strokes at the beginning of the session so that you prepare the muscles for the heavier techniques.

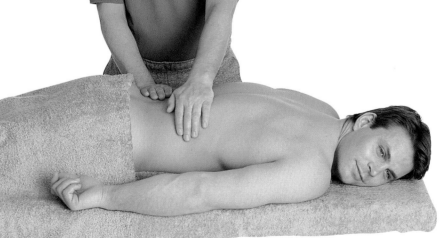

THE MASSAGE

1 Massage across the lower back, sliding your far hand toward you and the other one away from you. Keep your hands relaxed.

2 Now reverse the movement, sliding your hands in opposite directions. Repeat several times. Then place your hands slightly farther up the back, toward the middle, and carry out the same strokes. You can also massage over the pelvis and buttocks.

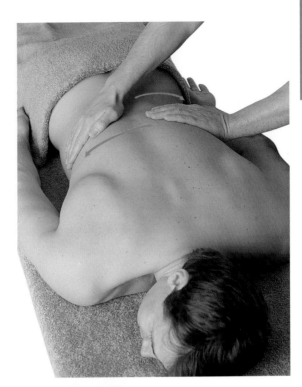

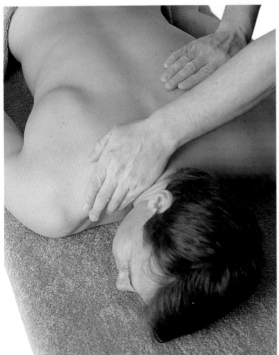

3 Once you have massaged the lower and middle back, continue the stroking toward the upper back. When you reach the upper back, slide your hands to include the shoulders.

4 You can repeat the same series of strokes as you work your way down the back toward the pelvis. Maintain a constant speed: the slower your movements, the more relaxing the massage.

WHOLE BACK: *Medium Stroke*

Applied with medium pressure, the strokes described here increase relaxation and enhance the circulation. They also have a warming effect on the muscles, preparing them for the deeper massage strokes later in the routine. When carrying out these movements, take care not to apply any pressure to the spine.

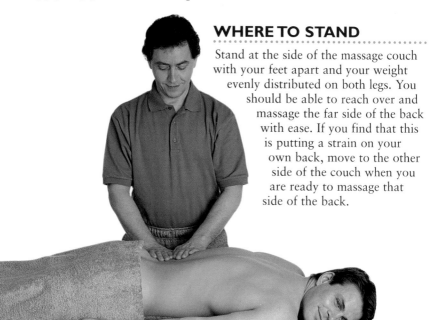

WHERE TO STAND

Stand at the side of the massage couch with your feet apart and your weight evenly distributed on both legs. You should be able to reach over and massage the far side of the back with ease. If you find that this is putting a strain on your own back, move to the other side of the couch when you are ready to massage that side of the back.

THE MASSAGE

Massage the lower back using both hands close together. Move them around in large circles, in a slow rhythm. Massage the side nearest to you first.

Option Instead of working on each side of the back separately, you can if you prefer use one large, circular movement to cover the whole of the lower back in one sweep.

I

2 Keeping your hands in contact with the back, reach over and repeat the same movement on the far side of the back. Accentuate the large, circular movements, as this action helps to increase the circulation in the local muscles and tissues. You can also increase the pressure by leaning forward with your body.

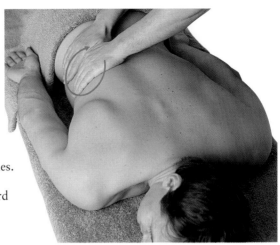

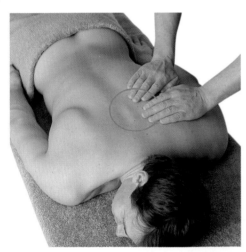

3 Repeat the same stroke on the upper back. To work on this area, move closer to the shoulders so that you can easily reach the whole of the upper back without putting any strain on your own back. Use small, circular movements to massage one side at a time.

Option If you prefer, you can use one large circular movement to massage the whole of the upper back and shoulders.

ONE-HANDED MASSAGE

You can also apply the same circular movement using only one hand. Although this may be more comfortable, you may find you are not able to exert as much pressure as you do when using both hands. Rest your free hand on the back while you massage with the other hand.

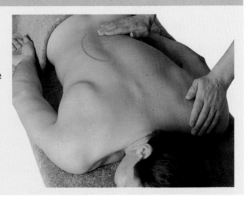

LOWER BACK: *Medium Stroke*

When you have warmed up the tissues by massaging them lightly, you can apply more concentrated pressure to the back. In addition to loosening the muscles, this massage sequence aids the local circulation of the back. The stroke is most valuable when the muscles are overworked, for example, after playing sports or doing some other strenuous physical activity.

WHERE TO STAND

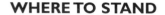

Stand close to the couch with your feet slightly apart and your weight evenly distributed on both legs. You may find it easier to stand with one foot slightly behind the other, as this means you can lean forward and increase the pressure of your hands. When stretching to reach the far side, take care not to strain your own back. You may prefer to change sides to massage the other side of the back.

Tight muscles

If the muscles of the person you are massaging are tense, some areas of the back may be slightly tender to touch. Provided the tenderness is not extreme, you can still massage these areas. Lean forward slightly in order to increase the pressure as you work the lower back; this will also help the circulation within the muscles. If this is painful for the person receiving the massage, discontinue it.

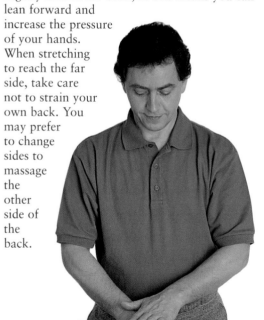

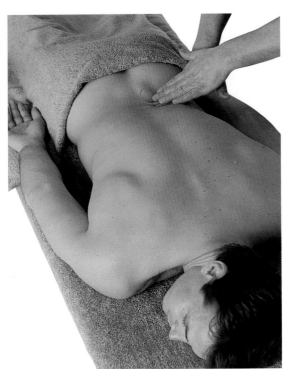

THE MASSAGE

1 Place the fingers of one hand on the side of the lower back nearest to you. Cover them with the fingers of the other hand to reinforce them.

2 Massage over the lower back using small circular movements, clockwise or counterclockwise. Use medium to deep pressure, and as you work keep your hands close to the spine where the main muscles are located.

3 Maintain a steady, slow rhythm with the circular movements, allowing your body to move with each stroke. If you can reach comfortably, continue the massage up into the middle back.

4 Reach over and massage the far side of the back. If this feels as if it is straining your own back, move to the other side of the couch. Use the same circular movements, small enough to concentrate the pressure on one section of the muscle group at a time. Avoid putting any pressure on the spine.

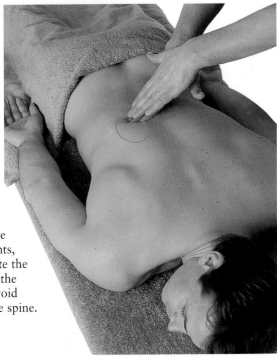

LOWER BACK: *Deep Stroke*

Bad posture and lack of exercise are common factors associated with tightness in the muscles, particularly in the lower back region. Deep massage strokes can help to relieve tightness in this area. Very little oil or cream is needed for this massage stroke.

ADJUSTING THE PRESSURE

- Always apply pressure gradually; it should never be heavy enough to cause pain.
  - Ask the recipient for feedback so you can adjust the pressure to a comfortable level.
  - As you work, increase the pressure on muscles that feel tight and knotted, and reduce it as tissues soften.

Warning!

Because of the amount of pressure involved, you should discontinue the massage if it causes any discomfort or pain. A person with sciatica or spinal problems should not have this massage at all.

WHERE TO STAND

Stand well balanced next to the massage couch with one foot slightly behind the other. Maintain as upright a position as possible and keep your working arm straight as you reach over to massage the other side of the back.

THE MASSAGE

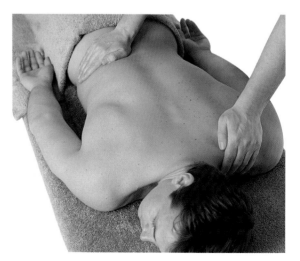

Place the heel of one hand on the far side of the spine, in the hollow of the back, but not on the spine itself. Bend the palm slightly so you can apply more pressure with the heel. Keep your fingers straight or curve them around the body's contours. Place your second hand farther up the back to support your weight.

2 Massage from the spine out, across the lower back muscles and down the side of the trunk. Apply most of the pressure with the heel of your hand. You can also lean forward slightly to increase the pressure through your arm.

3 Slide the heel of your hand forward to meet the fingers. Do this very slowly to allow sufficient force to reach the muscles and to reduce the chances of the hand slipping, then ease off the pressure.

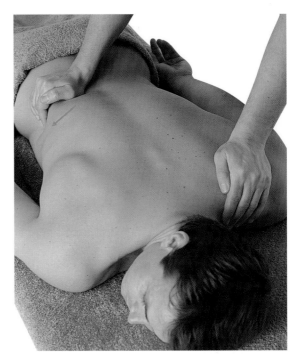

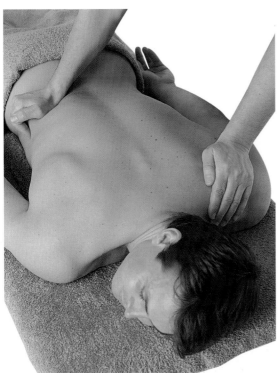

4 Repeat the same movement several times over the same area. Then place your hand slightly farther up the back toward the head, and repeat the routine. Do not place your hand on the lower rib cage as this area is close to the kidneys, which are best avoided.

5 Once you have completed the massage on one side, move around to the other side of the couch and repeat the movement on the other side of the back.

LOWER BACK: *Deep Stroke*

As an alternative or in addition to the one-handed stroke explained on pages 18–19, you can give deep-pressure massage with both hands. The chief benefit of this massage is that it stretches the muscles, which is particularly useful if they have become tense and knotted through overexertion, but it can also be used to improve circulation in the lower back. Because of the heaviness of the stroke, it is essential that you avoid the spine and that you reduce the pressure if the massage causes any discomfort or pain.

WHERE TO STAND

Stand next to the massage couch with your body facing the person you are massaging. You may feel more comfortable if you place one foot slightly behind the other to help your balance. Twist your trunk slightly so you can easily rest both hands on the lower back without overstretching your shoulders or elbows. You should not have to lean very far forward or impose any strain on your own back.

Warning!

If this stroke causes discomfort to the person you are massaging, reduce the pressure or discontinue it. It is important to avoid putting weight on the spine.

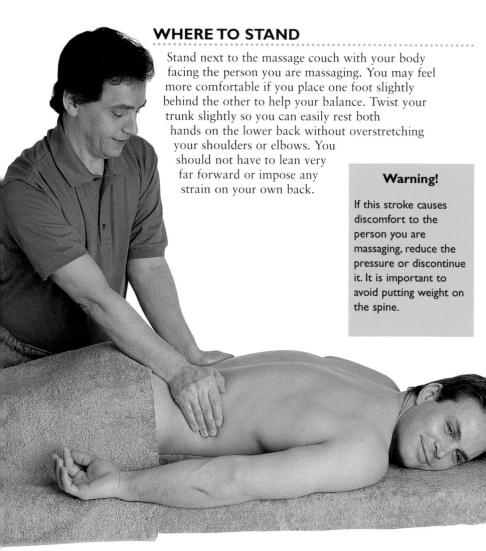

THE MASSAGE

1 Position your hands so that the heel of each one is close to the spine and the fingers are pointing out. The whole of each palm and all the fingers should be in contact with the skin surface. Lean slightly forward so you can exert some pressure through your arms, but take care that you do not apply any weight on the spine or rib cage.

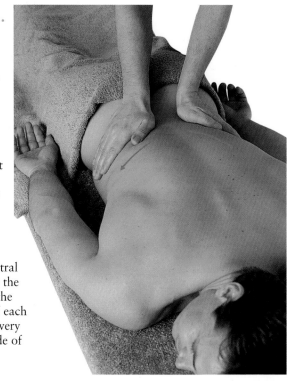

2 Massage from the central area of the back, near the spine, applying most of the pressure with the heel of each hand. Move your hands very slowly out toward the side of the trunk.

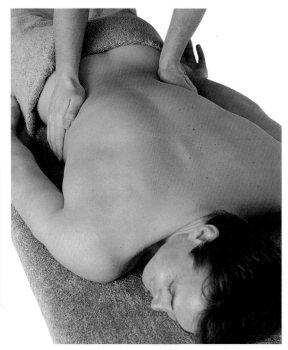

3 Curve your hands to follow the contours of the body. As you reach farther around to the side, toward the abdomen, reduce the pressure, then remove your hands.

4 Return to the central area of the back to repeat the movement. The person you are massaging should find the degree of pressure acceptable, and should experience the movement as a gentle, outward stretch of the muscles.

UPPER BACK: *Medium Stroke*

The muscles of the upper back are often tight or rigid, sometimes even more so than those of the lower back, and can therefore benefit a great deal from massage. A medium-pressure massage on the upper back area stimulates the local circulation and also promotes relaxation. The various strokes described in the following pages can be combined or repeated several times.

ALTERNATIVE

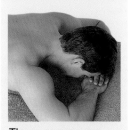

The person you are massaging may prefer to support his head on his hands or on a rolled-up towel. While the muscles of the upper back may not relax completely, this may be the only position in which the recipient feels comfortable.

WHERE TO STAND

Stand at the head of the massage couch with your feet slightly apart and your weight evenly distributed on both legs. Position yourself a slight distance from the couch so you are able to lean your whole body forward and exert pressure through your shoulders and arms.

Alternatively, stand with one foot slightly behind the other. You can apply pressure through your arms equally well from this position and may find that you are better balanced.

Make sure that whatever stance you adopt does not put a strain on your own back while you are performing the massage.

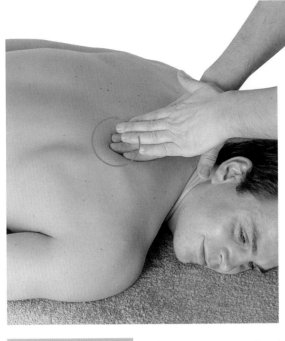

THE MASSAGE

1 Begin the massage on one side of the back. Use either hand, supporting it with the other hand. Work over the whole area using small, circular movements. For maximum benefit, repeat several times.

2 If you can reach it comfortably, also massage the middle of the back.

3 Now move your hands across to the other side of the upper back and repeat the same series of movements. Massage close to the spine, spending some extra time there if the muscles feel tight or knotted. Continue the circular movements to extend the massage over the shoulder blade (see box).

SHOULDERS

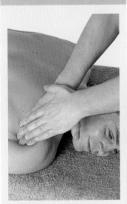

Massage over the bony shoulder blade area, using the same massage stroke but applying some extra pressure. Continue toward the shoulder and the upper arm.

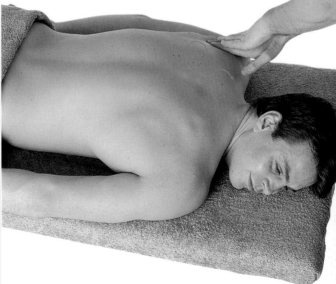

UPPER BACK: *Deep Stroke*

Once you have warmed up the muscles and tissues of the back with light and medium strokes, you can apply deeper massage to encourage further relaxation. To give the muscles time to relax fully, do not hurry the massage; increase the pressure gradually and only when the tissues offer less resistance. Take care not to apply too much oil or cream so that your hands do not slip.

ALTERNATIVE

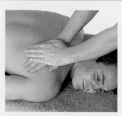

To exert more pressure on large or tight muscles, support one hand with the other. Work down one side of the spine at a time, then on each shoulder blade. Keep the pressure even, but increase it slightly when you reach very tight areas.

WHERE TO STAND

Stand at the head of the couch with one foot slightly behind the other so you can shift your body forward as you apply the massage stroke. You will need to bend forward slightly to massage the upper back, but keep this to a minimum to avoid straining your own back.

THE MASSAGE

I Place your hands at the top of the back, one on each side of the spine. Point your fingers toward the feet. Make contact with the heel of each hand, and keep your palms and your fingers flat.

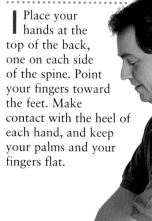

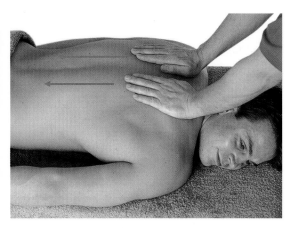

2 Press with the heel of each hand to massage the muscles on each side of the spine. Work from the top to the middle of the back, only as far as is comfortable. Return your hands to the upper back, and repeat the stroke several times. Do not massage over the spine itself.

3 Now place one hand on each side of the upper back, close to the spine. Massage over the shoulder blade and rib cage, working out toward the side of the trunk. Reduce the pressure slightly because the muscles here are not as bulky as those of the center back. Repeat the stroke a few times. Keep to a slow rhythm.

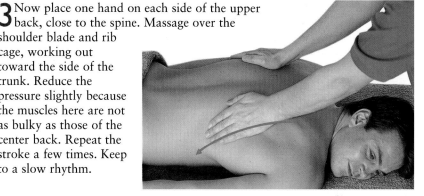

ALTERNATIVE

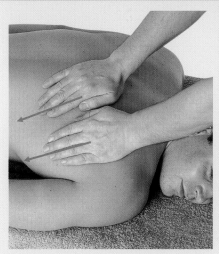

It may be more comfortable for you to apply the outward stroke using both hands close to each other. Massage one side of the back at a time. Start close to the spine and work toward the side of the trunk, sliding your hands over the shoulder blade and outer rib cage. Apply equal pressure with both hands, but less pressure than for the center back where the muscles are more bulky. Repeat a few times before moving to the other side of the back. You may find it easier to shift your body slightly to one side of the couch and then massage the opposite side of the back.

UPPER BACK: *Fist Massage*

If you use your fist, you can give a deep massage that exerts considerable pressure on very tight or knotted areas. Muscles that have been overworked also benefit, so this massage is especially useful after heavy physical activity or sports.

WHERE TO STAND

Ask the person you are massaging to rest his forehead on his hands. If this is not comfortable, he can turn his head to either side. Stand at the head of the massage couch with one foot slightly behind the other so you can lean forward and apply pressure. Alternatively, stand with your feet slightly apart and your weight evenly distributed on both legs.

MAKING A FIST

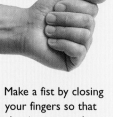

Make a fist by closing your fingers so that the tips are on the heel of your hand. The tips should be straight and not curled inside the palm.

THE MASSAGE

Place your fists on the upper back, one on each side of the spine, and lean forward to apply your body weight through your arms. Keep your back as straight as possible to avoid straining it.

2 Keeping your fists completely flat to the surface so that the knuckles do not dig into the tissues, massage slowly toward the middle back. Increase the pressure on tight areas and reduce it on areas that are more relaxed. Repeat several times.

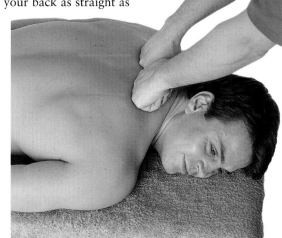

WHOLE BACK: *Cupping Stroke*

Cupping is a percussive-type movement that involves striking the tissues gently with the cupped hands. Although it is very invigorating and primarily used for toning the muscles, it can also be very relaxing. Cupping may be used at any time during a massage routine; however, it is mostly applied toward the end. You can start and finish the cupping movements anywhere on the back.

WHERE TO STAND

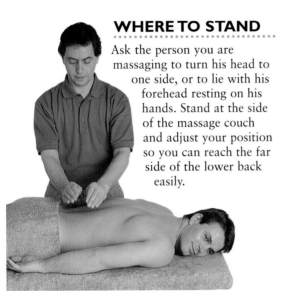

Ask the person you are massaging to turn his head to one side, or to lie with his forehead resting on his hands. Stand at the side of the massage couch and adjust your position so you can reach the far side of the lower back easily.

MAKING A CUP

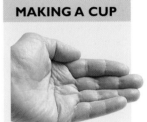

Without closing your fingers, curl your hand as if you were holding a small, round object. Keep your hand cupped throughout the movement, on and off the back.

THE MASSAGE

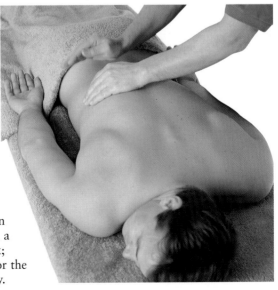

Strike the surface of the back with both hands alternately, striking with one as you remove the other. Apply light rather than heavy pressure, periodically checking that the pressure is acceptable to the person you are massaging. Do not apply this stroke to the spine or to the kidneys, in the region of the lower ribs. Maintain a steady rhythm as you work; cupping is more relaxing for the recipient if it is done slowly.

FINISHING BACK MASSAGE

This soothing, relaxing, featherlight stroke completes the massage routine on the back. It can also be applied between other strokes and even at the beginning of the massage routine for the back.

WHERE TO STAND

Stand next to the massage couch facing toward the head of the person being massaged. For this movement you will need to lean forward and reach the upper back, twisting your trunk slightly. This should not cause any strain to your own back; if it does, omit the first movement and use the strokes across the back instead.

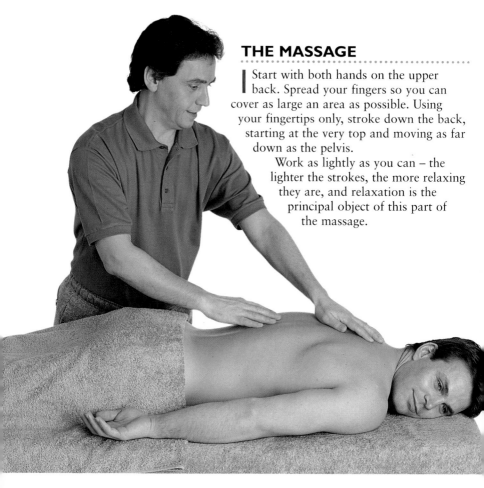

THE MASSAGE

Start with both hands on the upper back. Spread your fingers so you can cover as large an area as possible. Using your fingertips only, stroke down the back, starting at the very top and moving as far down as the pelvis.

Work as lightly as you can – the lighter the strokes, the more relaxing they are, and relaxation is the principal object of this part of the massage.

2 As you reach the lower back with the fingers of one hand, start to stroke from the neck downward with the other hand. Continue to alternate the strokes for a few minutes. Massage first one side of the spine, then the other. As long as the pressure is extremely light, you can also extend the stroking over the spine.

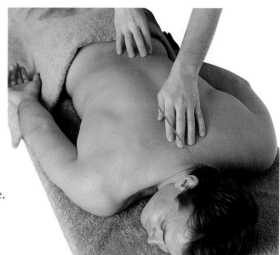

3 You can adapt the massage by taking your hands diagonally across the back. Use the same alternating strokes. Each stroke should be about 12 inches (30cm) long, but you can vary the length. Start at the far side of the back and work toward the side nearest you.

4 A further variation is to slide your hands transversely across the back. Start the stroke with one hand on the far side and massage across the back toward you. Alternate your hands using the same light, stroking movements.

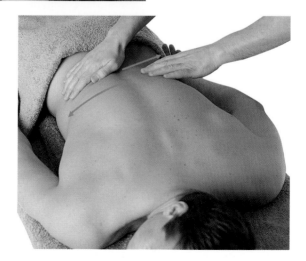

LOWER BACK: *Massage in Pregnancy*

Pregnancy is usually accompanied by an increase in weight, fluid retention, and impaired circulation. These physiological changes can contribute to the aching back that many women experience during pregnancy, particularly in the later months. Massage can help to soothe the general achiness, as well as promoting relaxation and improving the circulation of the whole back.

WHERE TO STAND

You may find it easiest to kneel for this stroke, or you may prefer to sit on a low stool or chair. You could sit on the floor, although this position may not allow you such good access to the upper back.

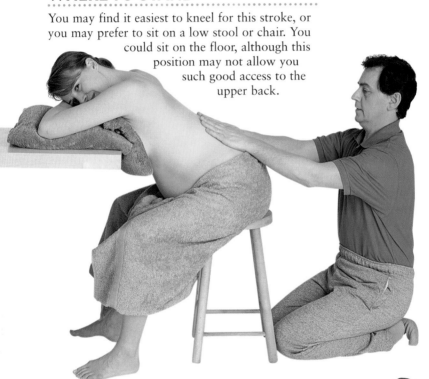

PREPARING A PERSON FOR MASSAGE

For massage a pregnant woman should sit in one of two ways.
■ She may sit on a chair or stool, with her arms resting on a table and her upper body and head supported by cushions and folded towels. It is essential that she is comfortable during the massage, so adjust the supports as necessary.
■ If there is no table, she may sit astride the chair, resting her folded arms on the back. This position may be more comfortable for her than resting her head on a table.

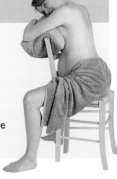

USING ESSENTIAL OILS

Some essential oils, made from the essences of herbs, flowers, and other substances, may not be suitable for use during pregnancy. It is therefore advisable to check about their safety when you make your purchase. The safest oils include camomile and lavender. Some authorities are now questioning the use of any essence on babies, even though these essences have been considered safe in the past.

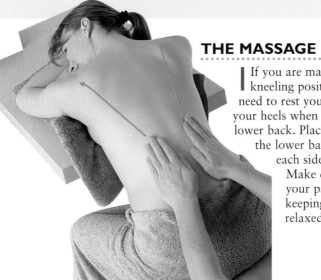

THE MASSAGE

I If you are massaging from a kneeling position, you may need to rest your buttocks on your heels when you massage the lower back. Place your hands on the lower back, one hand on each side of the spine. Make contact with your palms and fingers, keeping both hands relaxed.

2 Massage from the lower back up in the direction of the head. When you get to the upper back, slide your hands out, toward the shoulders.

3 Massage over the shoulders and then down the side of the trunk. Finish at the center of the lower back. Repeat the whole movement several times. Apply an even pressure, which should be firm but not heavy.

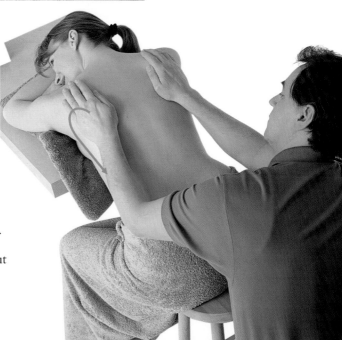

LOWER BACK: *Massage in Pregnancy*

The task of the muscles of the lower back, found alongside and fairly close to the spine, is to straighten the back and maintain an upright posture. During pregnancy they have to make postural adjustments, for example, to counteract the hollowing of the back that occurs during the later months. They also have to balance the posture and adjust to the extra weight carried at the front of the body. As a result, these muscles are more susceptible to tension and tightness than those of the upper back, and benefit from a heavy massage.

WHERE TO STAND

To perform the massage, kneel down on one or both knees. Place yourself at a distance from the woman you are massaging so you can easily lean forward. This helps you to transfer your body weight through your arms and increase the pressure of the massage.

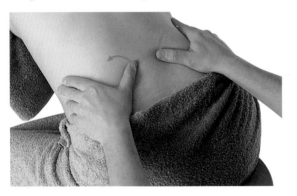

ALTERNATIVE

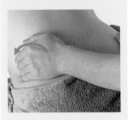

If you want to apply more pressure, perform the massage with the heel of each hand. To do this, you will need to position yourself slightly more to the side of the woman you are massaging. Work in small, circular movements, keeping your wrists fairly straight to avoid straining them. Concentrate on the central muscles near the spine.

THE MASSAGE

1 Place your thumbs flat on each side of the spine. Curve your palms and fingers around the back muscles and slightly to the side of the trunk.

2 Massage the muscles on each side of the spine by sliding the thumbs up and out, continuing each stroke for about 2 inches (5cm). Keeping the thumbs straight, apply pressure as you stroke up. Release it as you bring them down again.

3 When the muscles feel soft, move your hands up the back and repeat the strokes. Continue this way until you reach the middle of the back. Avoid any pressure on the spine.

The Legs

THE LEGS

One of the main benefits of leg massage is improved circulation. When the leg muscles contract, they squeeze the blood vessels and in so doing push the blood back up toward the heart. Leg massage compresses the vessels in a similar way, complementing the muscle contractions and assisting the flow of blood. Improved circulation also helps to relieve leg muscles that are tight and contracted due to strenuous physical work or exercise, or to anxiety. Overworking muscles leads to a buildup of metabolites (by-products of muscle contraction) and toxins; both can cause muscle fatigue. By increasing the circulation, massage helps to flush these out. Massage to the legs can also benefit arthritis sufferers, pregnant women, and anyone who has cellulite.

2

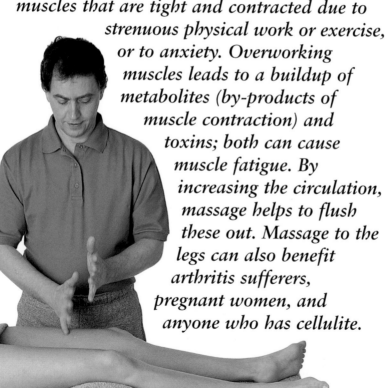

BACK OF THIGH: *Light Stroke*

L eg massage begins with a light and gentle stroke to relax the muscles and to improve the overall circulation. As in all other regions of the body, this type of stroke warms up the muscles and tissues in preparation for deep massage and prevents them from contracting when heavier pressure is applied.

WHERE TO STAND

Stand at the side of the massage couch with your feet slightly apart. Maintain an upright posture and keep your back more or less straight. If you find that you have to bend too much in order to place your hands on the thigh, spread your feet farther apart and lower your body.

Warning!

Do not massage the legs if a person has:

- varicose veins;
- sciatica, or pain down the back of the leg;
- excessive buildup of fluid in the lower leg;
- muscle tears which are severe and painful.

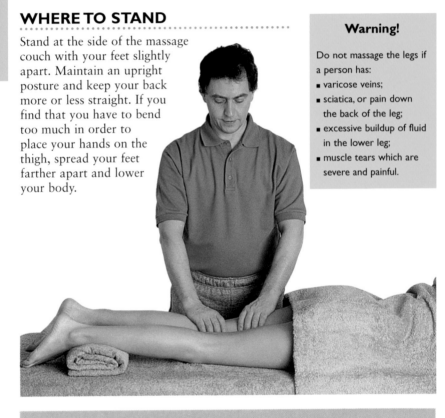

PREPARING A PERSON FOR MASSAGE

- The person being massaged should lie face down, with the head turned to whichever side is more comfortable.
- Place a flat cushion or folded towel under the abdomen to prevent unnecessary hollowing of the back. The feet should be supported with a cushion or rolled-up towel, placed under the ankle and the lower end of the shin bone. For extra comfort and support, a soft pillow or cushion may be set under the chest.
- The back should be covered with a towel to keep it warm during the massage.

THE MASSAGE

1 Place both hands on the back of the thigh, fingers pointing away from you. Relax your hands and curve them around the thigh. Start below the back of the knee and move upward; stop before your hands reach the buttock. Then lift your hands, return them down to the lower end of the thigh, and repeat several times.

2 Maintain a steady rhythm, allowing 3–5 seconds for the hands to reach the top of the thigh. Gradually increase pressure with both hands to enhance the circulation.

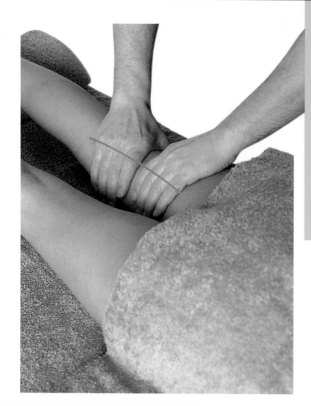

2

ALTERNATIVE MASSAGE

Alternate hands
Instead of massaging with both hands simultaneously, you can alternate the strokes. Massage with the right hand, from below the knee to the top of the thigh, then lift it off as you repeat the stroke with your left hand. Repeat a few times.

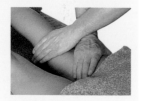

Massage with one hand
You may find it easier to do this movement using one hand instead of two, especially if the thigh of the person you are massaging is very slim. Start the massage just below the knee and work up toward the top of the thigh, varying the pressure depending on whether it is intended for relaxation or to improve the circulation. Lighter pressure tends to be relaxing while heavier pressure improves the circulation.

BACK OF THIGH: *Deep Stroke*

S tretching the muscles at the back of the thigh (the hamstrings) can be an ongoing challenge, because these muscles are often tight. Regular exercise is often required in this situation. Massage is also beneficial, providing a further stretch of the muscle fibers.

WHERE TO STAND

Stand at the side of the massage couch. You may find it easier to carry out this movement if you stand with one foot slightly behind the other, so that you are well balanced. Alternatively, stand with your feet next to each other and slightly apart, and with your weight evenly distributed between them.

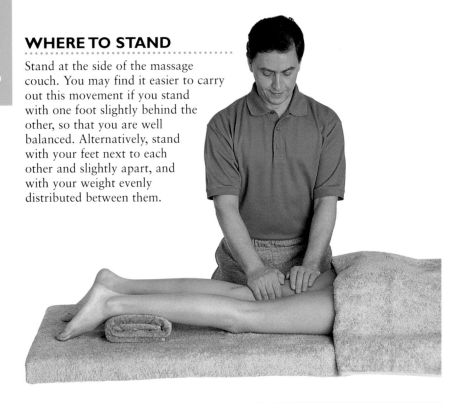

MUSCLE TIGHTNESS AT THE BACK OF THE THIGH

■ Restriction or muscle hardness is sometimes called fibrotic tissue. This may be caused by tightness brought on by a lack of exercise; it is even more likely to be the outcome of prolonged periods of sitting. Difficulty in touching the toes may be a sign of tightness in these muscles.

■ Scar tissue buildup is another cause of restriction. Buildup usually results from repeated straining of the muscles.

■ A substantial muscle tear can also create temporary muscle spasms. Massage should be applied only when the healing is complete.

2

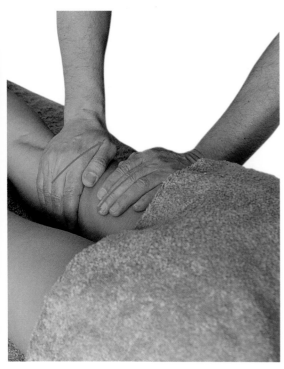

1 Place both hands side by side on the back of the thigh. Let your palm and fingers relax and curve around the thigh muscles. Start with the right hand on the inner side of the thigh and the left hand on the outer thigh.

2 Push your hands in opposite directions, the right hand outward and the left one inward. As you massage, apply some deep pressure in order to squeeze the muscle.

3 When you reach the outer edge of the thigh, stop squeezing the muscles. Then massage back across the thigh, again squeezing the muscles as you progress. At the end of this sequence, your hands will finish where they started.

4 Continue the strokes a few times on one part of the thigh, then move the hands to another section and repeat.

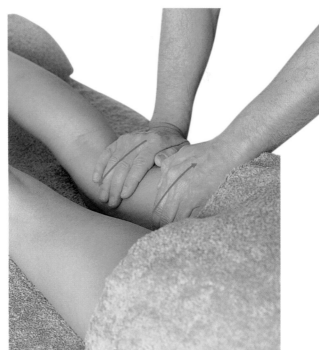

BACK OF THIGH: *Toning Stroke*

Hacking and cupping are percussive (tapping) strokes which are used to tone and warm up bulky muscles. They can be used to help prepare the legs for strenuous activity such as sports, or included in the massage routine for the thigh. Follow the percussive movements with a light massage similar to that carried out at the beginning of the thigh routine (see pp. 34–35). If the person you are massaging suffers from severe muscle weakness, varicose veins, cellulite, or sciatica, these strokes may cause discomfort and should be left out.

WHERE TO STAND

Maintain your standing position at the side of the massage couch. Keep your back fairly straight when you apply the toning strokes. Aim also to relax your shoulders as well as your arms throughout the movement.

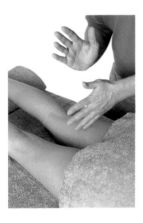

HACKING

Position your hands so the palms face each other and the little fingers are close to the thigh. Spread the fingers of each hand and, using a flicking action of your wrist, strike the thigh with your little finger. Quickly lift your hand, spreading the fingers open again. Now strike the thigh in the same way with your other hand.

    Continue with this alternating action of both hands over one section of the muscle group for a few seconds, then move your hands to another position and repeat the action.

CUPPING

Without closing your fingers, form your hands into cup shapes by tightening them as if you were holding an object such as a small ball in each hand. Keep the hands in this position as you lightly strike the muscles, alternating your hands. Cover the whole surface area of the thigh in this way. Maintain a steady rhythm: a slower speed is more pleasant and relaxing for the person receiving the massage than a faster one.

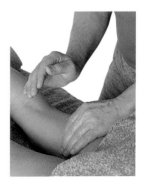

CALF MUSCLE: *Light Stroke*

As with the thigh and other parts of the body, the routine for the calf starts with a light massage, followed by deeper techniques. Most, if not all, massage movements are soothing to some degree, but these light strokes are the most effective method of inducing relaxation. They are also of great value because in some cases they are the only ones that can be tolerated by the person receiving the massage.

WHERE TO STAND

Stand to the side of the massage couch, close to the calf of the person you are massaging. Avoid leaning forward when you place your hands on the calf muscles. If you find this difficult, lower your body by spreading your feet apart and bending your knees if necessary.

ALTERNATIVES

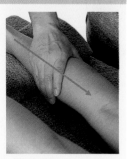

You can vary the massage by using only one hand. Place one hand parallel to the recipient's calf. Rest your other hand on her thigh. Massage from the lower calf toward the thigh. When you reach the back of the knee, remove your hand and return it to the lower calf. Repeat this light stroking movement several times.

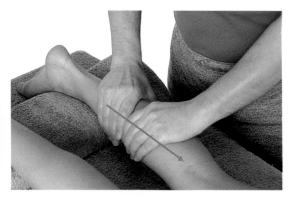

THE MASSAGE

Place both hands across the calf, with the fingers pointing away from you. Curve the palm and fingers around the shape of the calf. Keep your hands close to each other as you slide them along the calf. Massage from the base of the calf toward the back of the knee, taking a few seconds to complete the stroke. Apply an even but very light pressure. Remove your hands and return them to the base of the calf. Repeat several times.

You can alternate which hand you use. Massage with the right hand first, then remove it when you reach the back of the knee and start the massage with the left hand.

CALF MUSCLE: *Medium Stroke*

A medium massage is used to assist the circulation in the lower leg. It also helps reduce any buildup of fluid (edema), especially around the ankle. The amount of pressure used for these movements has to be adjusted according to the effect you are trying to achieve. A very light massage will help reduce fluid buildup; a slightly heavier one is more effective at enhancing the circulation. Both are also relaxing.

2

CIRCULATION IN THE LOWER LEG

- Poor circulation in the lower leg is often due to lack of exercise and long periods of standing.
- Pregnancy is also frequently associated with circulation problems of the lower legs, caused by extra weight and lack of overall mobility. This often results in muscle cramps and spasms.
- Bad circulation causes congestion in the veins and surrounding tissues. A common feature of congestion is the formation of varicose veins. These are a source of pain and discomfort which are exacerbated by touch.
- Fluid retention around the ankle is another feature of poor circulation.

Warning!

It is not safe to apply this massage to the lower leg if the person you are massaging suffers from severe conditions such as a heart problem, or from varicose veins.

WHERE TO STAND

Stand at the foot of the massage couch, facing the head of the person you are massaging. You may find it easier to have one foot slightly behind the other. Shift your body weight on to your front foot as you move your hands toward the knee. Then shift it onto the back foot as you take your hands down toward the ankle area. Support the ankle on a rolled-up towel.

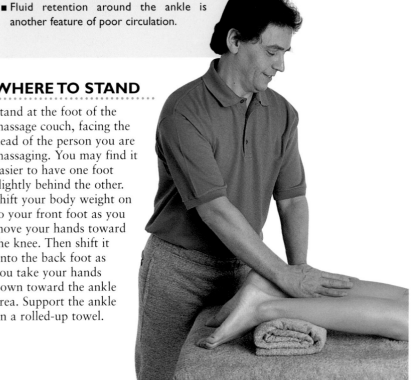

THE MASSAGE

1 Place one hand on each side of the calf, with the palm and fingers parallel to the muscles of the lower leg. Start with the hands just above the ankle and massage up toward the thigh. Continue the stroke to the back of the knee or to the lower thigh. Then remove your hands or slide them to the lower calf again.

2 Repeat the short massage stroke over the calf a few times. Apply equal pressure with the palm and fingers of both hands and reduce the pressure as you go over the back of the knee.

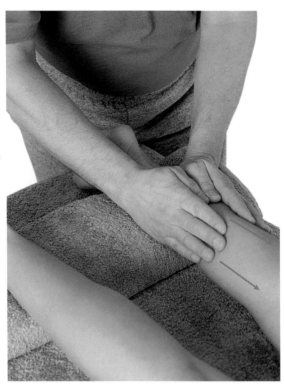

2

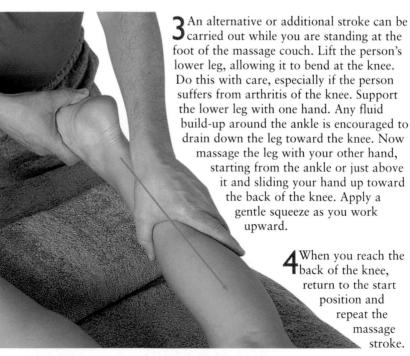

3 An alternative or additional stroke can be carried out while you are standing at the foot of the massage couch. Lift the person's lower leg, allowing it to bend at the knee. Do this with care, especially if the person suffers from arthritis of the knee. Support the lower leg with one hand. Any fluid build-up around the ankle is encouraged to drain down the leg toward the knee. Now massage the leg with your other hand, starting from the ankle or just above it and sliding your hand up toward the back of the knee. Apply a gentle squeeze as you work upward.

4 When you reach the back of the knee, return to the start position and repeat the massage stroke.

CALF MUSCLE: *Deep Stroke*

Muscle tightness in the calf can be reduced with the stretching and compression action of this movement. In addition, the squeezing action of the massage helps the circulation in the muscles and reduces congestion in the lower leg.

WHERE TO STAND

Position yourself close enough to the side of the massage couch to enable you to place your hands on the recipient's calf without straining your back. Place your hands on the calf so they lie across the muscles, with the fingers on the inside of the calf and the thumbs on the outside.

THE MASSAGE

1 Apply a gentle squeeze with the fingers and thumb of each hand. Compress the muscles in this way with both hands simultaneously. Maintain your gentle grip on the muscles and lift them up gently to stretch their fibers.

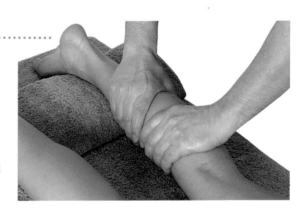

2 Hold the stretch for a few seconds, then release your grip completely, but without removing your hands from the legs. Repeat the squeezing and lifting action several times along the whole length of the calf.

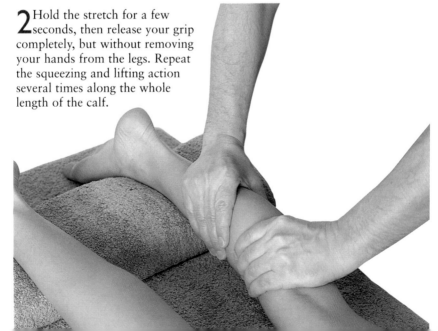

CALF MUSCLE: *Toning Stroke*

Toning massage to the calf muscles involves percussive movements such as hacking and cupping. They can be used for their stimulating effect – for example, before strenuous muscle work when participating in a sport. You can also include them in the general massage routine for the leg. Because they are heavy strokes, they should not be given to anyone with varicose veins or sciatica. Follow these toning movements with some light stroking (see p. 39) to soothe nerves and muscles.

2

WHERE TO STAND

Maintain the same standing position next to the massage couch. Lean forward slightly to apply the massage stroke. Alternatively, lower your body by spreading your feet apart and bending your knees.

HACKING

For this technique, place your hands so the palms face each other and the little fingers are close to the calf muscles. Spread your fingers out and strike the muscles with the little finger. Remove your hand by flicking the wrist, at the same time striking the tissues with the other hand in the same way. Continue to alternate the hands for a few seconds on one area. Then repeat the movement over the rest of the calf.

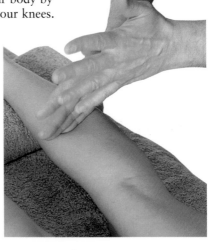

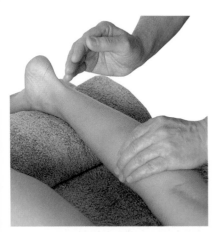

CUPPING

To perform the technique known as cupping, half-close your hands into a cup shape. Gently strike the tissues with one hand in this position; the action should produce a hollow sound. As one hand lifts up, strike the same area with the second hand. Continue with this alternating striking action for a few seconds and then move to another area of the calf, until you have covered the whole region. Use only light pressure and keep to a slow rhythm.

THE FEET: *Squeezing*

The feet work extremely hard, and yet they are often the most neglected part of the body. Foot massage is therefore a well-earned treat and, despite some common apprehensions, can be surprisingly enjoyable. However, the feet are very sensitive and will always be, for some people, an area not to be touched.

WHERE TO STAND

For this stroke you need to be standing at the foot of the massage couch. Give yourself enough space that you can easily alternate the stroking with each hand. Keep your back straight throughout the movement and avoid rounding your shoulders as this will put undue pressure on them.

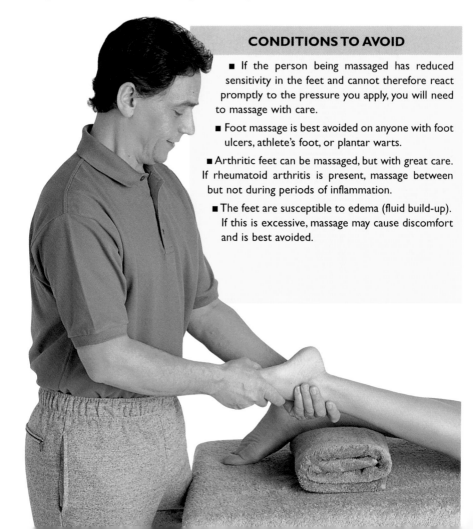

CONDITIONS TO AVOID

■ If the person being massaged has reduced sensitivity in the feet and cannot therefore react promptly to the pressure you apply, you will need to massage with care.

■ Foot massage is best avoided on anyone with foot ulcers, athlete's foot, or plantar warts.

■ Arthritic feet can be massaged, but with great care. If rheumatoid arthritis is present, massage between but not during periods of inflammation.

■ The feet are susceptible to edema (fluid build-up). If this is excessive, massage may cause discomfort and is best avoided.

THE MASSAGE

1 Slowly lift the lower leg, allowing it to bend at the knee. Put one hand under the ankle to support the lower leg, with fingers underneath and thumb on top. Grip the ankle gently, especially if there is any tendency to edema. Raising the lower leg encourages fluid to drain from the ankle toward the knee, so it is of benefit if there is any congestion around the ankle.

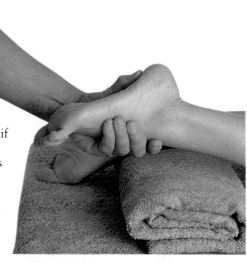

2

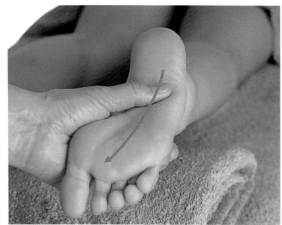

2 With your fingers underneath and your thumb on top, gently squeeze the foot. Maintain this grip as you slide your hand toward and over the toes.

3 As your hand nears the toes, support the foot at the ankle with your other hand. Repeat the same action of squeezing and sliding your other hand toward the toes. Continue with this alternating massage for a minute or so. This is a particularly relaxing stroke, so be prepared to continue it for a while if the person you are massaging wishes it.

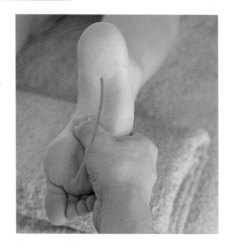

THE FEET: *Relaxation*

In addition to fatigue, the feet often suffer from inefficient circulation. As a result they may frequently be cold, with the toes particularly affected. These massage movements are pleasant and soothing as well as being very beneficial for the overall circulation.

WHERE TO STAND

Continue to stand at the foot end of the massage couch. In order to place your hands comfortably on the foot, you may need to lower your body by bending your knees slightly. In this posture you can avoid having to bend forward and the possibility of straining your back.

THE MASSAGE

1 Fold both your hands around the ankle and heel of one foot, with your fingers on top and your thumbs on the sole. Keep the foot resting on the cushion, and squeeze it with the fingers and thumbs of both hands.

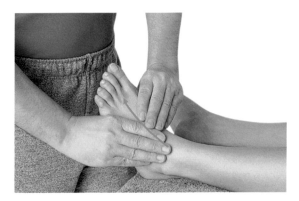

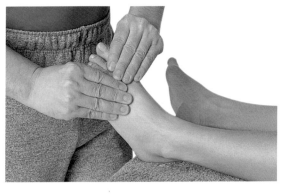

2 Slide your hands toward the toes, keeping the same grip all the way. When you reach the toes, release the pressure and return your hands to the ankle. Repeat the stroke several times. As you work upward, you may also lift the foot slightly.

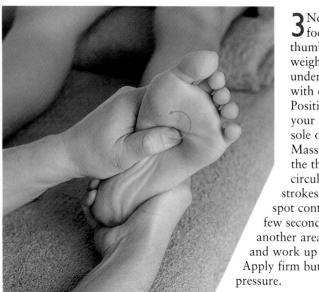

3 Now massage the foot with your thumbs. Support the weight of the foot, underneath the heel, with one hand. Position the thumb of your other hand on the sole of the foot. Massage the sole with the thumb, using circular or straight strokes. Massage one spot continuously for a few seconds, then move to another area. Start at the heel and work up toward the toes. Apply firm but comfortable pressure.

2

4 You can use the other hand to perform the same thumb massage on the sole of the foot and the toes. Massaging the toes can be slightly awkward due to their small size. If you find this a problem, it may help to support the toes by placing your fingers behind them as you massage with your thumb. Use light, even strokes.

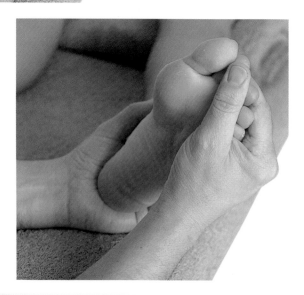

REFLEX POINTS

Organs and different parts of the body are reflected in corresponding points on each foot through connecting energy pathways. These points are known as reflex points. It is likely that a nervous connection also exists between the organs of the body and the feet. Massage on the sole of the foot may cause some discomfort on the reflex points, but this should decrease as the massage progresses.

THE FRONT LOWER LEG

The muscles at the front of the lower leg are used extensively in activities such as bicycling, tennis, and running. This massage stroke is of great benefit for those who partake in these sports. Apart from being relaxing and pleasant, it assists the circulation within the lower leg muscles. It is also of help in conditions where congestion builds up in the lower leg and ankle, for example, in pregnancy.

2

WHERE TO STAND

This medium-stroke massage to the lower leg can be carried out while you stand at the foot of the massage couch or at the side. If you stand at the foot, you can lean forward slightly to increase the pressure of your stroke. Standing at the side allows for a gentler and perhaps a smoother stroke.

THE MASSAGE

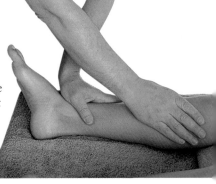

1 Start the massage on the lower leg using only one hand. When you reach the knee, follow with the other hand. Without applying too much pressure, massage from the ankle to the knee. Continue over the knee itself, but reduce the pressure on this area. Then remove your hand and place it on the ankle again. Repeat the alternating strokes a few times.

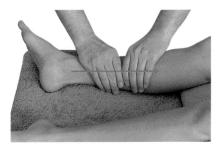

2 The same stroke can be carried out from a position at the side of the massage couch. Curve your hands across the leg, with your fingers pointing away from you. Massage with both hands simultaneously, starting at the ankle and working up to the knee. Reduce the pressure as you go over the knee.

Option Alternate your hands instead of moving them together. Apply one stroke with one hand and follow with the other. Do not pause between strokes; try to achieve a continuous movement.

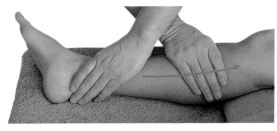

THIGH FRONT: *Medium Stroke*

This massage for the front of the thigh continues the work of improving the circulation. Like all other strokes for circulation, this massage is also used for relaxation. In addition, it helps to prevent congestion, such as that associated with varicose veins and cellulite.

WHERE TO STAND

To massage the thigh, stand to the side of the couch and face the head of the person you are massaging. Place one foot slightly in front of the other. Shift your weight onto the front foot as you move your hands up the thigh, then onto the back foot as you return them to the knee area. Avoid too much twisting of your trunk.

2

THE MASSAGE

1 Place your hands close together on the thigh, one on each side and just above the knee. Keep each hand flat against the skin surface. Use some pressure as you massage with both hands over the front and sides of the thigh, working up toward the pelvis, but stopping before you reach the groin.

2 Lift your hands or slide them gently back toward the knee. Repeat the movement several times.

ALTERNATIVE

An alternative method for massaging the thigh is to use one hand instead of two. This allows you to use the hand closest to the massage couch, keeping any twisting of your trunk to a minimum.

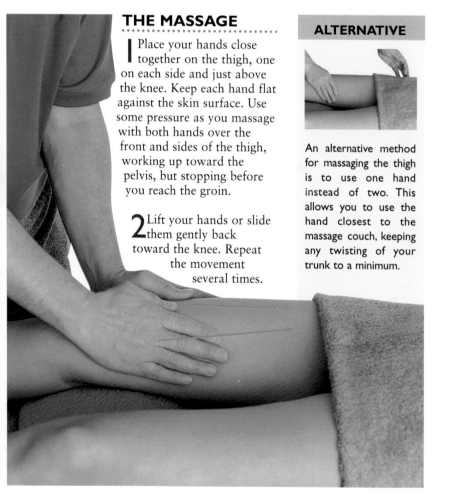

THIGH FRONT: *Deep Stroke*

In addition to the relaxation strokes, this deep massage is used on the thigh muscles to relieve tension by stretching the muscle fibers and to reduce any buildup of metabolites, the by-products of muscle work. Because of the deep pressure involved, this massage may not be suitable on muscles that are very weak or sensitive.

WHERE TO STAND

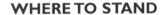

For this movement you will need to place your hands on the middle of the thigh of the person you are massaging and exert some pressure. This means that you will need to twist your trunk slightly and at the same time reach over the thigh. Avoid any uncomfortable position that might put a strain on your back. If you cannot do this stroke comfortably, it is better to leave it out. It may be more comfortable for you to carry out this movement while sitting on the edge of the massage couch. You may not exert as much pressure as when you are standing, but the movement is equally pleasant.

ALTERNATIVE

If you are carrying out the massage on the floor, you may find it easier to perform this stroke while kneeling astride the leg you are massaging. From this angle you will find you can apply considerable downward pressure onto the thigh muscles. Control the movement so that it is even, to avoid any accidental slipping of the hands.

2

THE MASSAGE

1 Place the heels of both hands close to each other at the center of the thigh, with your fingers curving around the thigh and pointing in opposite directions. Your hands should be positioned on the belly of the muscles, midway between knee and groin. Apply pressure with the heels of your hands by leaning forward slightly.

2 As you increase the pressure, the heels will sink into the muscles. Slide your heels outward, maintaining the same pressure, in order to stretch the muscles across their fibers.

3 When you reach the outsides of the thigh, ease off the pressure. Lift your hands and return them to the front of the thigh. Repeat the stroke several times on the same area, then move your hands to another position farther up or down the thigh and repeat the series of strokes. The amount of pressure you apply should always be comfortable for the person being massaged.

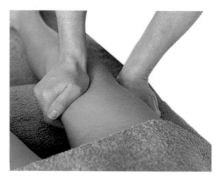

CELLULITE

- Cellulite is a condition in which fat is trapped within tiny, fibrous capsules near the surface of the skin.

- The condition is caused by congestion, poor circulation, an imbalance of electrolytes (such as sodium and potassium) and an accumulation of fat. A hormone imbalance may also be a contributing factor to cellulite.

- Once cellulite is established, it is difficult to reverse. Improved circulation plus dietary changes can go some way to preventing or improving the condition. In addition to massage, exercise can be used to reduce congestion by enhancing the circulation of blood and fluid (lymph). Daily brushing of the skin with a natural bristle brush also helps to lessen the congestion.

THIGH FRONT: *Toning Stroke*

These massage strokes, using techniques known as hacking and cupping, tone the muscles of the front of the leg. Apart from their general stimulating effect, they are a pleasant addition to the massage routine for the leg. The main muscles that benefit from this toning massage are those on the front of the thigh and those on the outer side.

2

WHERE TO STAND

Stand a slight distance away from the side of the massage couch so you can carry out the toning strokes with ease. You may find it easier to lower your body by bending the knees slightly. Aim to have your forearms more or less horizontal, as for the other toning strokes.

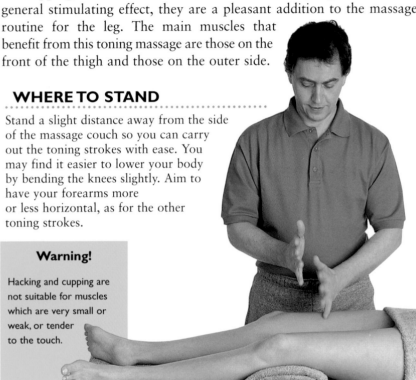

Warning!

Hacking and cupping are not suitable for muscles which are very small or weak, or tender to the touch.

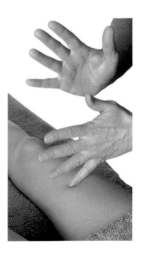

HACKING

1 Place your hands over the thigh just above the knee. Have your palms facing each other, your fingers spread, and the little fingers close to the skin surface. With a flick of the wrist, strike the thigh muscles with the little finger of one hand, allowing the other fingers to cascade onto the little finger. Immediately lift your hand and at the same time strike the muscles with the other hand.

2 Repeat this hacking movement with alternate hands over the whole area. Concentrate on the main muscles on the front and outer side of the thigh and ease off the pressure when you reach the inside of the thigh.

CUPPING

I Cup each hand by curling the palm and fingers. Line up both hands on top of the muscles, with the fingers pointing away from you. Strike the thigh with one cupped hand. As you lift this hand, bring down your other hand.

2 Continue with this alternating stroke for a few seconds. Then move your hands to another section and repeat the same series of strokes. Cover the front of the thigh and outer muscles; ease off on the inside.

PICKING UP

I Picking up is another toning movement. Place your hands next to each other across the thigh, with the thumbs on the outside and the fingers on the inside. Squeeze the muscles and tissues gently between the fingers and thumb of one hand.

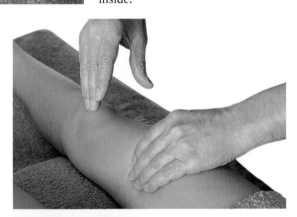

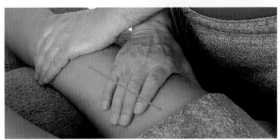

2 At the same time lift the tissues up and slide your hand off, then immediately repeat the squeezing and lifting action with the other hand. Continue over the whole thigh region.

FINISHING

Complete the toning routine with a soothing massage (above). Place your hands across the thigh, with fingers and palm flat on the surface. Without using any pressure, massage from the knee to the upper thigh. Slide both hands together or alternate them. Do not pause between strokes; make the massage one continuous stroking action. Repeat several times.

THE WHOLE LEG

A featherlight massage completes the routine on the entire front of the leg. It helps soothe the muscles and nerves following all the other massage movements. The lightness of the touch combined with a very slow rhythm promotes a deep sense of tranquility throughout the whole body.

WHERE TO STAND

Position yourself facing the head of the recipient so you can reach the top of the thigh and the ankle comfortably; if necessary lower your body by spreading your feet and bending your knees.

2

ALTERNATIVE

An alternative method of carrying out this massage is to stand facing across the massage couch. In this position you can apply the massage stroke using both hands together instead of alternating them.

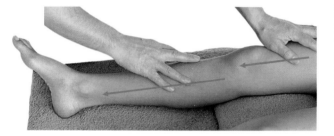

THE MASSAGE

I Start with one hand on the upper thigh. Spread your fingers and rest the fingertips on the thigh. Drag the fingers gently over the skin, working down to the ankle.

2 When you reach the lower leg, start the same movement from the top of the thigh with the other hand, so that the hands follow each other down the leg.

3 Finish each stroke at the ankle, then lift your hand and return it swiftly to the upper thigh. This makes the massage continuous, with no pauses between strokes. Do not hurry the movements or apply any pressure: the weight of your hands is enough.

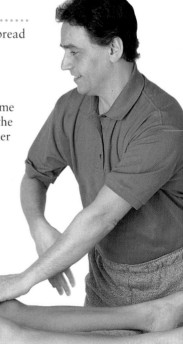

The Abdomen and Chest

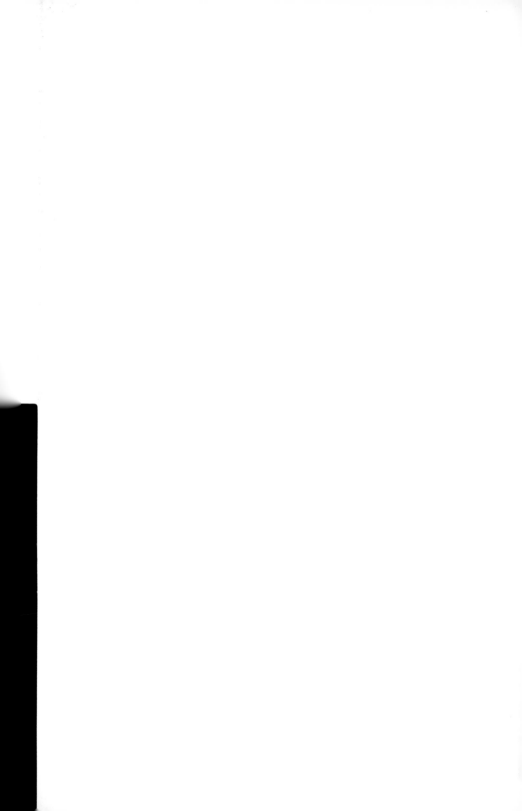

THE ABDOMEN AND CHEST

Abdominal massage promotes deep tranquility, which in itself helps to improve the functioning of the digestive system. It assists the forward movement of the contents of the intestines and improves the function of the organs by enhancing their circulation. By warming the tissues, massage also helps to break up fatty deposits in the abdominal wall. Chest massage eases those muscles involved in breathing, particularly when these are overworked. It also reduces any tightness or restricted movement in the rib cage.

3

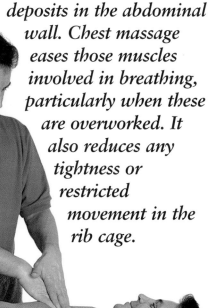

THE ABDOMEN: *Light Stroke*

The massage routine for the abdomen begins with a gentle movement, performed slowly with very light pressure in order to promote relaxation. It is important to use a gentle contact in this region as the abdomen is very sensitive, and even the lightest touch can cause the abdominal muscles to contract. Although muscle contraction is a normal protective reaction, it can be exacerbated by tension. In cases of severe anxiety, massage to the abdomen may be tolerated better at the end of a whole body massage when the recipient has had time to relax.

CAUTION
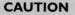

- Avoid abdominal massage if there is any pain, tenderness, or discomfort.
- Do not massage the abdomen soon after a meal.
- Abdominal massage is best avoided in the early months of pregnancy.
- Menstrual cramps can make the abdomen too painful to massage.

3

WHERE TO STAND

Stand close to the massage couch, with your feet slightly apart and your body weight distributed evenly on both legs. Your forearms should be more or less horizontal and your hands flat on the surface of the skin and relaxed. Aim to keep your back straight, bending forward only slightly as you reach over to massage the far side of the abdomen.

PREPARING A PERSON FOR MASSAGE

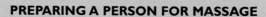

For massage to the abdomen and chest, the following posture should be adopted:
- The person you are massaging should lie on his back, with a cushion under his head and his legs covered with a towel.
- To relax the stomach muscles and make the massage easier to carry out, ask the person to bend his knees and support them on a cushion or rolled-up towel.
- To reduce any tension that may be held within the abdomen, apply a mild heat pack, such as a moist, hot towel, before the massage.

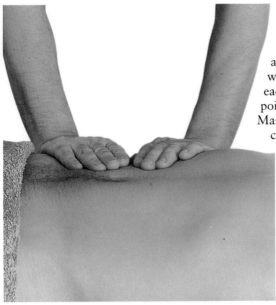

THE MASSAGE

1 Place your hands on the side of the abdomen closest to you, with the thumbs next to each other and the fingers pointing away from you. Massage in a large clockwise circle that follows the flow of the contents of the large colon. Very little pressure is needed: the weight of your hands is sufficient. Keep a steady and slow rhythm, taking about five seconds to complete one circle.

3

2 As you massage over the central area of the abdomen, slide your upper hand (the one nearest to the chest) over the lower part of the rib cage. This helps to increase the circulation to the diaphragm and to the muscles between the lower ribs.

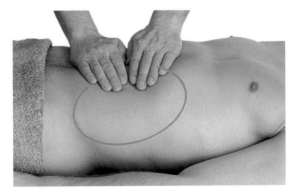

3 Then reach over to the farthest side of the abdomen, curving your hands around the abdomen until they touch or almost touch the couch on the opposite side. Continue massaging in a circle over the central abdominal area or the lower part of the abdomen. Finish the massage on the side nearest to you. Repeat the same circular stroke several times.

THE ABDOMEN: *Medium Stroke*

A medium massage is now performed on the central abdominal area. The aim of this stroke is to reduce tension in the muscles and to enhance the general circulation within the abdomen, and also to encourage dispersal of the fat that is often abundant in this region.

3

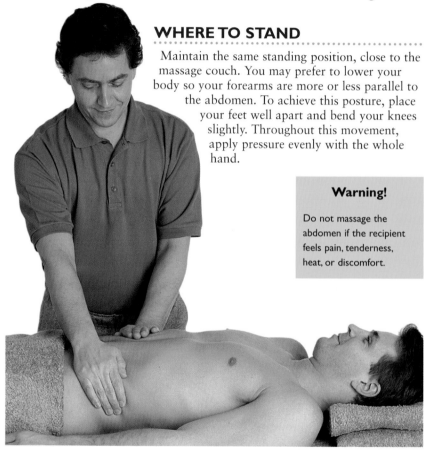

WHERE TO STAND

Maintain the same standing position, close to the massage couch. You may prefer to lower your body so your forearms are more or less parallel to the abdomen. To achieve this posture, place your feet well apart and bend your knees slightly. Throughout this movement, apply pressure evenly with the whole hand.

Warning!

Do not massage the abdomen if the recipient feels pain, tenderness, heat, or discomfort.

THE MASSAGE

I Place one hand on the far side of the abdomen and the other hand on the side nearest to you. Point the fingers of both hands away from you.

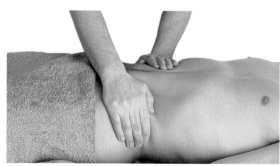

2 Keeping your hands relaxed and applying an even pressure with your palms and fingers, slide the far hand toward you and push the closer one away from you. As you move toward the center of the abdomen, squeeze the muscles and tissues (including fatty tissue).

3 Release your hold as you continue to slide your hands to the outer edges of the abdomen. At the end of this movement, your hands will have crossed to opposite sides of the abdomen.

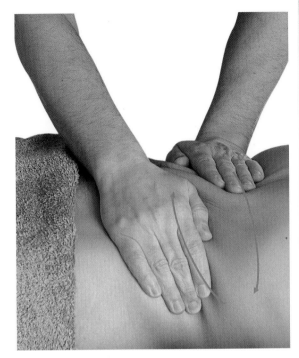

3

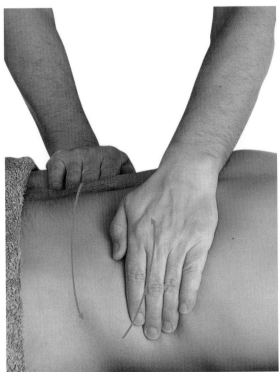

4 From this position, slide the hands across the abdomen once again and repeat the same squeezing action to the muscles and tissues.

5 When both hands are back at the starting position, carry out the whole movement several more times.

Remember: the abdomen is very sensitive, so always keep the pressure light, and introduce any slight increase very gently. Be guided by the reaction of the person you are massaging.

THE ABDOMEN: *Deep Stroke*

This deep massage has a number of benefits. It enhances the circulation within the digestive organs, which require a good supply of blood for optimum functioning. It encourages the forward motion of the contents of the intestine, alleviating such problems as constipation. And it helps the abdominal muscles to relax.

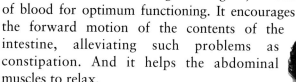

WHERE TO STAND

Stand at the side of the massage couch with your feet slightly apart and your weight distributed evenly on both legs. You should aim to keep your shoulders and arms relaxed as you apply gentle pressure with your fingers.

3

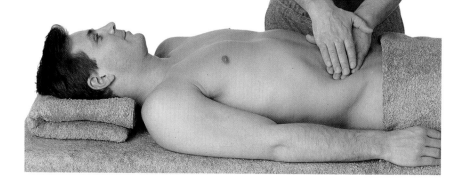

EFFECTS ON INTERNAL ORGANS

■ Massage to the abdomen helps the digestive organs by increasing their blood supply which in turn improves their function.

■ Massage also benefits the small and large intestines by physically assisting the forward movement of their contents.

■ Gurgling sounds can often be heard during the massage, indicating a healthy and active colon.

■ Massage can improve kidney function, which helps with the elimination of toxins.

THE MASSAGE

1 Place one hand on top of the other. Apply pressure with the upper hand. Move both hands together, clockwise or counterclockwise, in circles about 4 inches (10cm) in diameter. Increase the pressure at the start of the movement so the fingers of the lower hand sink into the tissues.

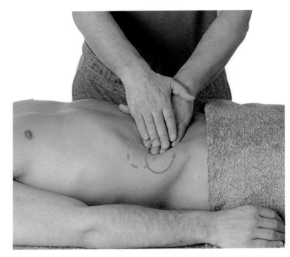

2 Release the pressure entirely before you complete the movement, and momentarily remove your hands from the surface of the abdomen. Make contact once again and apply the same circular massage, increasing the pressure as before, in particular on areas that feel tight. Reduce the pressure immediately if it causes discomfort.

3

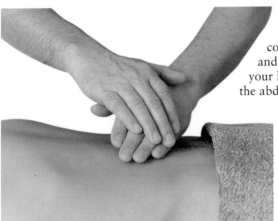

3 Repeat the circular massage in the same area a few times. Then move to another section and repeat the same routine. Continue in this way until you have massaged the whole abdomen. Remember that a deeper massage can be applied on the central area, which is more muscular, than on the outer areas of the abdomen.

WHOLE TORSO: *Light Stroke*

For a massage over the whole of the abdominal and chest area, use this continuous stroke with minimal pressure. If you are massaging a man with a hairy chest, you may need extra cream or oil. If you are massaging a woman, you should avoid the breasts.

3

Warning!

Avoid chest massage if the person you are massaging has:
■ a cold or flu
■ bronchitis
■ a heart problem
■ chest problems

WHERE TO STAND

To massage the abdomen and chest, stand at the side of the massage couch and face the head of the person you are massaging. Maintain a fairly upright and relaxed posture as you move your hands up the chest and in the direction of the shoulders.

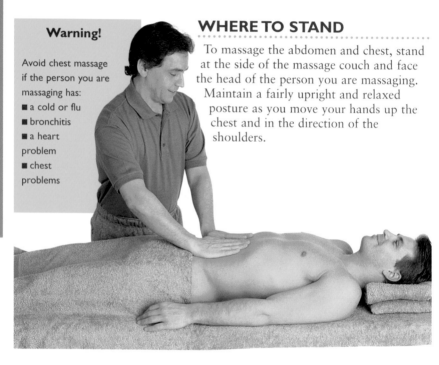

THE MASSAGE

Place your hands next to each other on the abdomen. Keep them relaxed and make contact with the palms and fingers. Slowly massage from the lower abdomen up toward the head.

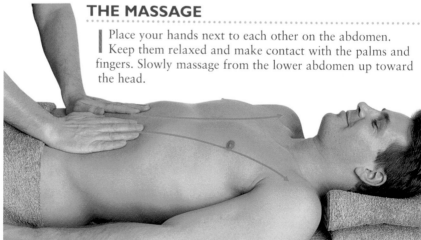

2 As your hands reach the upper chest, slide them outward toward the shoulders. Move your hands at the same slow speed and continue to apply the same light pressure. Cup your hands slightly to massage over the shoulders.

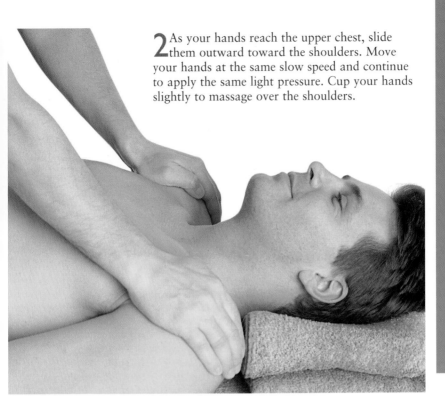

3

3 Continue down the outside of the trunk, then bring the hands back to the center of the abdomen. Repeat the stroke. Use the lightest pressure throughout, and reduce it immediately if it causes any discomfort.

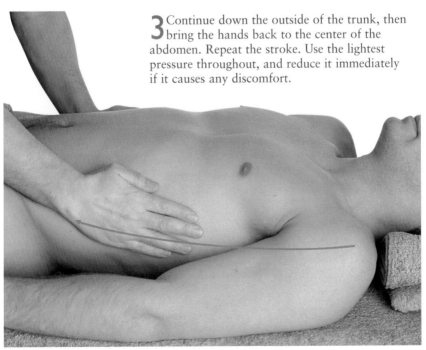

THE CHEST: *Medium Stroke*

Compared to other areas such as the back, the upper chest may not seem an area that needs massaging, yet it contains muscles that are used in several ways and which are often rigid and fatigued. These muscles, commonly known as the "pecs" but properly called the *pectoralis major* and *pectoralis minor*, extend as far as the collar bone and the arm. This massage helps to increase the circulation within the chest and these associated muscles. It is also relaxing and warms up the tissues in preparation for deeper massage work.

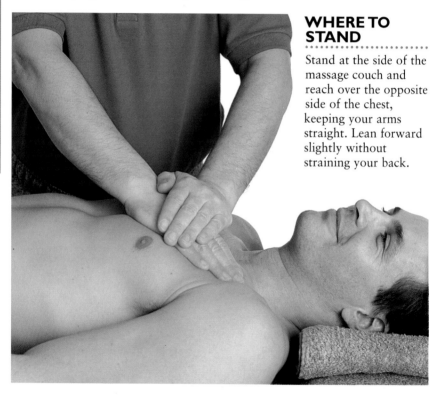

WHERE TO STAND

Stand at the side of the massage couch and reach over the opposite side of the chest, keeping your arms straight. Lean forward slightly without straining your back.

THE UPPER CHEST MUSCLES

The muscles of the upper chest – the "pecs" – are involved with all shoulder and arm movements and therefore in any form of physical work and sports. Some, particularly the upper chest muscles, have a key function in the mechanism of breathing. Others, such as those in between the ribs, play a similar role. Overuse, tension, or problems with posture cause the upper chest muscles to contract continuously. As a result, they often become fatigued and shortened. When this happens, breathing can be restricted.

THE MASSAGE

1 Place one hand on top of the other on the upper chest. Lean forward to apply some pressure from your shoulders through your arms. Massage out toward the shoulders. You should avoid massaging near the nipples.

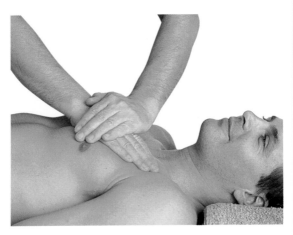

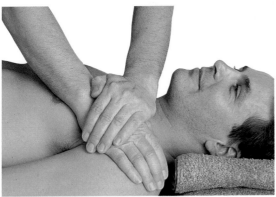

2 Continue the massage over the shoulder area following the direction of the muscle fibers. Cup your hands to massage around the shoulder. Then lift your hands or slide them back to the central area. Repeat the same massage stroke several times.

3

CHEST MASSAGE FOR WOMEN

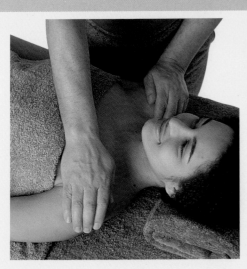

If you are massaging a woman, it is best to use only one hand as this produces less pressure and makes it easier to maneuver around the chest and avoid the breasts. Massage from the center of the chest up toward the shoulder, then cup your hand to go over the shoulder. Repeat the stroke several times. If the woman is menstruating or breastfeeding, the entire chest area can be quite tender, in which case you should perform the massage with the utmost care or, if it causes discomfort, omit it altogether.

THE CHEST: *Deep Stroke*

Deep massage on the upper chest muscles encourages further relaxation and loosens the muscles. Although you are applying deep pressure, you should adjust it to the state of the muscles, which can vary in size and tightness. Similarly, the duration of the massage must reflect the degree of tension in the muscles.

WHERE TO STAND

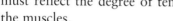

Stand at an angle to face the person you are massaging or position yourself in line with his shoulder. You may need to bend your elbow slightly in order to place both hands on the near side of the chest, and straighten them when you reach over to work on the opposite side.

3

THE MASSAGE

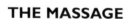

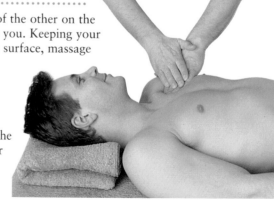

Place one hand on top of the other on the side of the chest nearest you. Keeping your fingers flat against the skin surface, massage around in small circles, clockwise or counter-clockwise, applying even pressure with both hands. Repeat these strokes a few more times. Then perform the same movement on another area until you have covered the whole of the chest area closest to you.

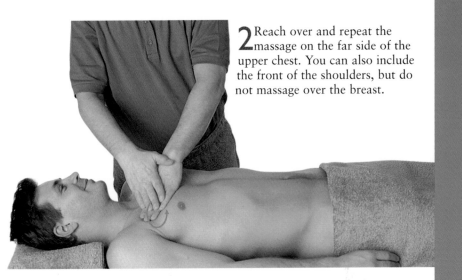

2 Reach over and repeat the massage on the far side of the upper chest. You can also include the front of the shoulders, but do not massage over the breast.

ALTERNATIVE POSITION

An alternative arrangement for massaging the upper chest is to stand at the head of the massage couch. Place one hand on top of the other and massage the area, using small, circular movements. Lean forward slightly to increase the pressure. Then repeat over the other side of the chest.

3

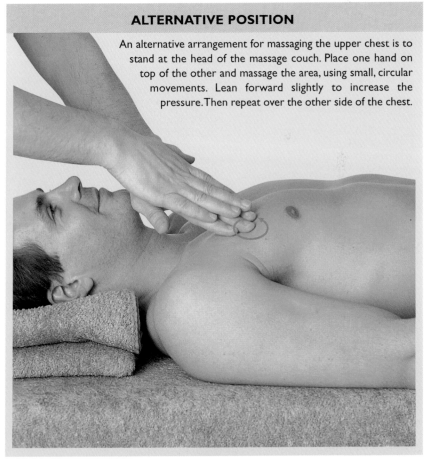

FINISHING THE MASSAGE

The massage routine for the abdomen and chest finishes with this light stroking movement over the upper chest. Since it is a relaxing stroke, it can be repeated several times.

WHERE TO STAND

Stand at the head of the massage couch, with one foot slightly behind the other. As you reach down the chest with your hands, shift your body forward without bending too much.

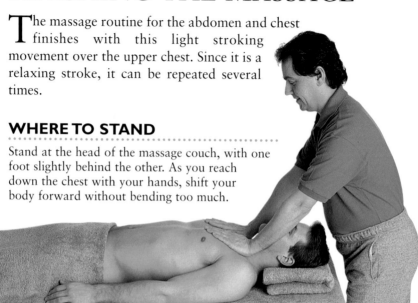

3

THE MASSAGE

1 Place your hands close together, on the central area of the upper chest. Make contact with the fingers and palm of each hand and keep both hands relaxed. Massage with both hands together, from the upper chest down toward the abdomen in long smooth strokes. There is no need to go over the abdomen itself, but go as far down as is comfortable. If you are massaging a woman, move your hands downward between the breasts toward the abdomen.

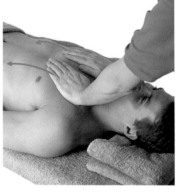

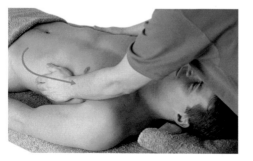

2 When you reach the abdomen or slightly before, continue the stroke outward from the center of the body to the outer edges of the rib cage. Still applying a light pressure, massage back upward toward the shoulder. Bring your hands back to the center of the upper chest and repeat the routine.

The Arms

4

THE ARMS

Poor circulation in the arms is unusual, but can lead to pain. The hands, however, are susceptible to poor circulation and often become cold as a result. Massage is highly effective in assisting the circulation of the whole arm, and of the hand in particular. Arthritic conditions in the shoulder, in the elbow, and more often in the hand can also cause pain in the arm. In some cases, very light, gentle massage soothes some of the pain. Nerve irritation or poor circulation caused by neck or shoulder problems can lead to "referred pain" in the arm. This is best treated by a specialist such as a physiotherapist or an osteopath. So too are problems relating to sporting activity, such as tennis elbow, or trauma. Massage can, however, be used for general relaxation and to soothe overused muscles.

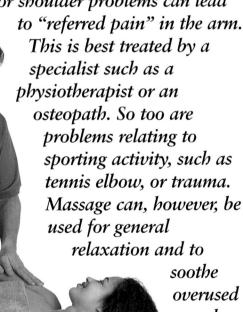

4

THE HAND: *Medium Stroke*

Almost anyone can benefit from a hand massage, whatever their age or state of health. The skill needed to massage the hand is instinctive and requires little effort. In addition to being very relaxing, hand massage improves the circulation and can help to soothe the pain of arthritis.

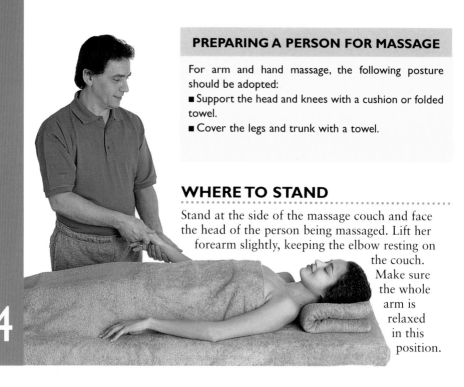

PREPARING A PERSON FOR MASSAGE

For arm and hand massage, the following posture should be adopted:
■ Support the head and knees with a cushion or folded towel.
■ Cover the legs and trunk with a towel.

WHERE TO STAND

Stand at the side of the massage couch and face the head of the person being massaged. Lift her forearm slightly, keeping the elbow resting on the couch. Make sure the whole arm is relaxed in this position.

4

THE MASSAGE

Use one of your hands to support the hand you are massaging. With the thumb of your free hand, massage the back of the person's hand, using small, circular strokes. Repeat several times over one area, before moving to another area. Use firm pressure, adjusting it as necessary to suit her level of tolerance. This massage is intended to be soothing, so it should not be vigorous or cause any discomfort.

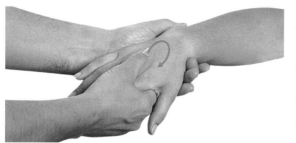

2 Massage the fingers one at a time. Squeeze each finger between your thumb and fingers, and simultaneously slide along the finger in one stroke, finishing at the tip. Release your grip, return to the first position and repeat the squeezing and sliding action.

3 To massage the palm, apply a series of small, circular strokes with your thumb all over the area. There are a number of small and yet very strong muscles in this region that will benefit from a fair amount of pressure.

4 Carry out all of the movements on one arm, then move to the other side of the person receiving the massage and repeat the strokes.

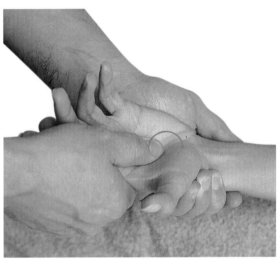

4

ARTHRITIC CONDITIONS

Some arthritic conditions, such as rheumatoid arthritis, are accompanied by episodes of inflammation and severe pain in the joints of the hands. It is not safe to apply massage until the inflammation has completely subsided, and even then only gentle massage is advisable. Other forms of arthritis, including osteoarthritis, may cause little inflammation. In these cases it is safe to carry out massage, though again it should be gentle and should be discontinued if it causes pain.

THE FOREARM: *Light Stroke*

This very pleasant and relaxing stroke combines a massage of the forearm and the hand. Although it is primarily a soothing stroke, it also benefits the circulation. The squeezing action involved promotes the arterial flow of blood toward the hand. As a result, any feeling of having cold hands is prevented or lessened.

WHERE TO STAND

Stand at the side of the massage couch and face the head of the person being massaged. Position yourself close to the arm so you can easily reach down to the elbow area.

4

THE MASSAGE

Bend the arm of the person you are massaging at the elbow, and wrap your hands around the forearm, near the elbow. Gently squeeze the arm as you massage with both hands upward, toward the wrist. If you are leaning forward and putting strain on your back, raise the arm by putting a folded towel under the elbow.

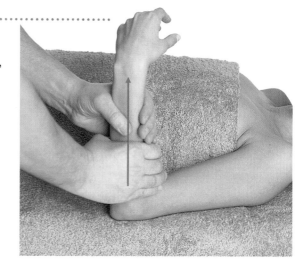

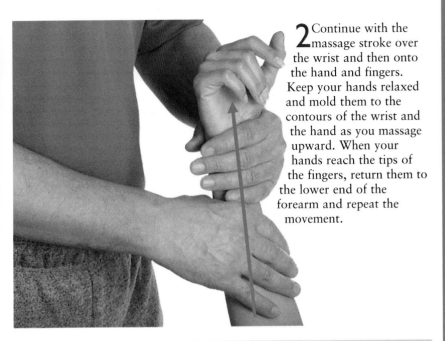

2 Continue with the massage stroke over the wrist and then onto the hand and fingers. Keep your hands relaxed and mold them to the contours of the wrist and the hand as you massage upward. When your hands reach the tips of the fingers, return them to the lower end of the forearm and repeat the movement.

ALTERNATIVE MASSAGE

If you are massaging someone with very slim forearms, you can use one hand instead of two to perform the massage. Support the hand of the person you are massaging with one hand and perform the massage with the other. Raise the arm up if necessary by supporting the elbow on a folded towel. Raising the arm prevents you from having to bend forward.

This arrangement can also be used as a simple alternative to the two-hand hold. Carry out the same stroke, starting at the elbow and working up to the fingers using either hand.

4

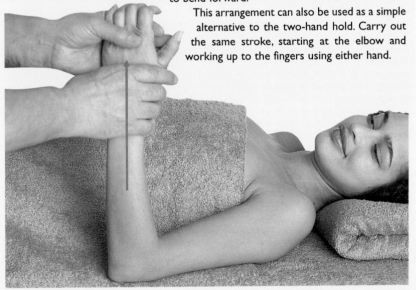

THE FOREARM: *Medium Stroke*

This medium massage to the forearm follows the direction of the venous flow (the blood flow through the veins) toward the heart. Its main benefit is that it improves the circulation; however, it also has a relaxing effect and fits in well with the massage routine for the arm.

ALTERNATIVE

As the arm is easy to massage, the person receiving the massage can be sitting instead of lying down. This may be more appropriate if the person you are massaging is elderly or not feeling well.

WHERE TO STAND

Maintain the standing position to the side of the massage couch. Raise the forearm slightly by bending the person's arm at the elbow. Aim to maintain an upright posture throughout the massage.

4

THE FOREARM MUSCLES

The hand, wrist, and forearm are inextricably linked in terms of the work they do; every movement of the hand and the wrist involves one or more of the several muscles of the forearm. It follows that this muscle group is used almost constantly, even more so during physical work and in sports. As a result, they are likely to be the tightest muscles in the arm. They are also susceptible to strain and injuries such as tennis elbow. Massage can help to reduce any tightness and maintain the stretch of the muscles, thereby preventing injury.

THE MASSAGE

Hold the wrist with one hand. Use your other hand to massage the forearm. Make contact with your palm and fingers, and apply gentle pressure. Start at the wrist and slide your hand as far as the elbow.

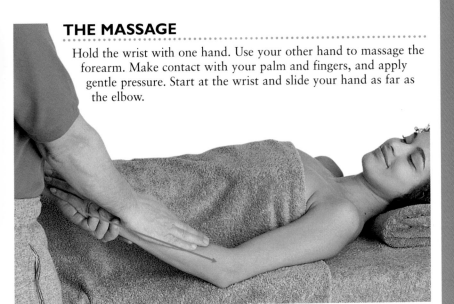

ALTERNATIVE POSITION

You can also massage the forearm at the same time as applying a gentle squeeze. Continue to hold the wrist with one hand, and place the thumb of your other hand on the outside of the forearm and the fingers on the inside. Squeezing gently, slide your fingers and thumb from the wrist toward the elbow. When you reach the elbow, remove your hand or slide it down to the wrist again. Repeat the stroke a few times. Keep the elbow of the person you are massaging on the couch throughout the movement.

4

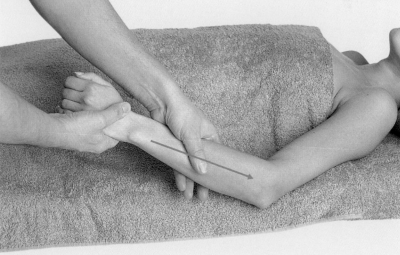

THE FOREARM: *Deep Stroke*

This deep massage improves the circulation of the forearm muscles and eases tension. As it also loosens the muscles and stretches them, it prevents the occurrence of injuries such as tennis elbow. The massage focuses primarily on the forearm muscles close to the elbow. Those nearer to the wrist are not big enough to be squeezed in this way.

TENDER MUSCLES

Muscles that are very tight may be a little tender when palpated. This movement therefore may cause some discomfort initially, until the muscles begin to relax and their fibers are stretched. If necessary, revert to some of the lighter massages given earlier in this chapter and work very gently until you feel the tight muscles loosening under your hands. If there is a strain, such as a tear in the muscle, any tenderness will be more severe and aggravated by this massage. This stroke, therefore, is best omitted.

WHERE TO STAND

Position yourself close to the massage couch so that you can easily bend the person's arm at the elbow and hold the forearm in an upright position. In order to avoid too much bending forward, you may want to raise the arm by placing a folded towel or cushion under the elbow.

THE MASSAGE

1 To massage the inner forearm, support the wrist with one hand and wrap the fingers of your other hand around the forearm. The heel of your hand should be on the inside of the arm.

2 Squeeze the forearm, applying most of the pressure with the heel of your hand. Roll the muscles toward your fingers, sliding the heel of your hand forward.

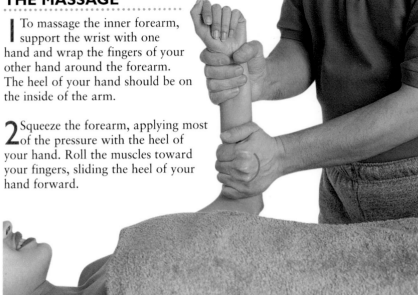

3 As you near the wrist, ease the pressure to avoid pinching the skin. Repeat a few times. Then massage the outer forearm. Hold the forearm at the wrist with one hand. Place your other hand near the elbow, with the fingers on the inside of the forearm and the heel on the outside. This is where the main muscle group is located and most of the pressure is applied.

4

4 Apply the same squeezing and rolling action as before. Repeat the action a few times.

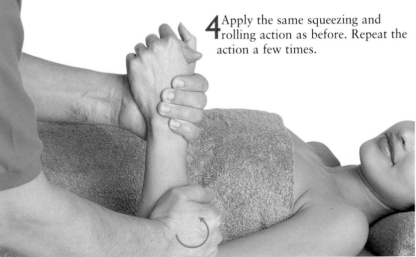

UPPER ARM: *Medium Stroke*

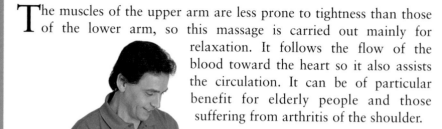

The muscles of the upper arm are less prone to tightness than those of the lower arm, so this massage is carried out mainly for relaxation. It follows the flow of the blood toward the heart so it also assists the circulation. It can be of particular benefit for elderly people and those suffering from arthritis of the shoulder.

WHERE TO STAND

Stand at the side of the massage couch and raise the arm to be massaged by supporting it with one hand at the elbow. Use the other hand to apply the massage stroke.

4

THE MASSAGE

1 Support the elbow with one hand and place your other hand just above the elbow. Keep your fingers and palm flat against the skin surface and your thumb close to your palm and index finger.

2 Slide your hand up toward the shoulder, still keeping it flat. Lean forward slightly and apply a little pressure with your hand.

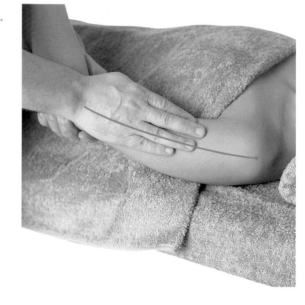

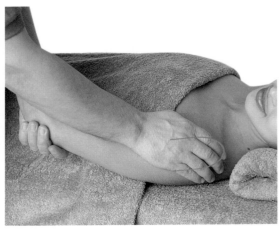

3 When you get to the shoulder, cup your hand to massage around the shoulder area. Then flatten your hand again and massage lightly down to the elbow. Repeat the same routine several times more.

ALTERNATIVE POSITION

Some of the massage strokes, including those of the upper arm, can be carried out with the person you are massaging sitting on a chair instead of lying on the massage couch. Make sure you are sitting or standing at a comfortable height and close to the person you are massaging. Avoid bending awkwardly or leaning forward too much as this can strain your back. You may find that massaging while you sit down is better than standing.

Use the same method of stroking, from the elbow up to shoulders. Massage the shoulder with your cupped hand and then flatten the hand to travel down to the elbow again. Repeat the same stroke several times.

4

UPPER ARM: *Deep Stroke*

Although the upper arm muscles are not usually tense or tight, they can be fatigued and overused from physical work and sports. This massage is used for relaxation and to loosen up this muscle group. It is of particular use on muscles such as the biceps when these are very large and developed.

WHERE TO STAND

Stand at one side of the massage couch. You will need to twist your trunk slightly in order to position your hands parallel to the upper arm you are going to massage. If this feels uncomfortable, reposition your hands so they lie more or less across the upper arm. You may find it easier to carry out this movement, and a number of other ones, too, sitting on the edge of the massage couch. A further adjustment is raising the level of the upper arm by placing a cushion or folded towel underneath it. The forearm of the person you are massaging can then rest on their abdomen. This is particularly useful if you remain in the standing position.

4

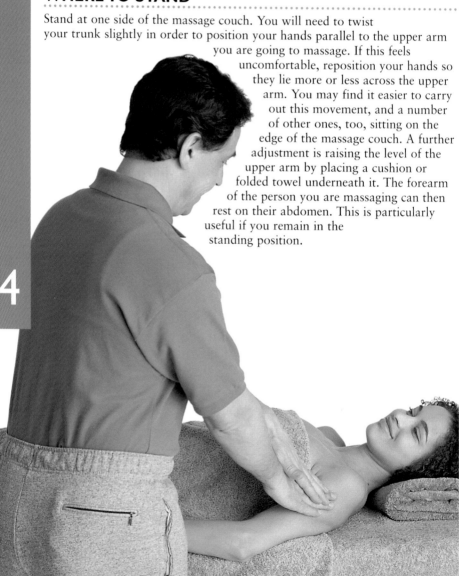

THE MASSAGE

1 Place your hands, one on top of the other, at the lower end of the upper arm, near the elbow. (The right hand can be on top of the left or vice versa, whichever is more comfortable.) Use both hands to carry out the massage and apply the pressure at the same time.

2 Using small circular movements, apply pressure as you move your hands around. Then ease the pressure slightly as you complete the circle. Repeat the stroke on the same area a few times.

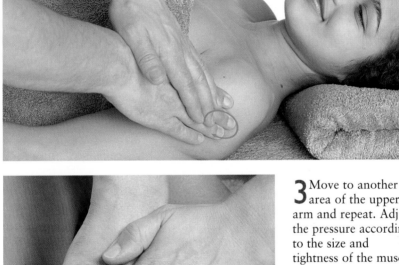

3 Move to another area of the upper arm and repeat. Adjust the pressure according to the size and tightness of the muscle group: the larger they are, the heavier the pressure needed. Make sure the level of pressure you are applying is acceptable to the person you are massaging.

4 Continue the massage over the whole of the upper arm, including the outer part of the shoulder.

4

FINISHING ARM MASSAGE

The massage routine for the upper arm ends with this featherlight movement. The purpose of the stroke is to soothe the muscles, tissues, and nerves. Like other featherlight strokes, it deepens the state of relaxation not only of the arm but also throughout the whole body. It is performed in a slow rhythm, with each stroke taking about 5 seconds to complete.

WHERE TO STAND

Position yourself so you can reach the shoulder area without bending forward too much. The massage stroke finishes at the wrist and hand, so you need to adjust your posture so you can also reach this area with ease.

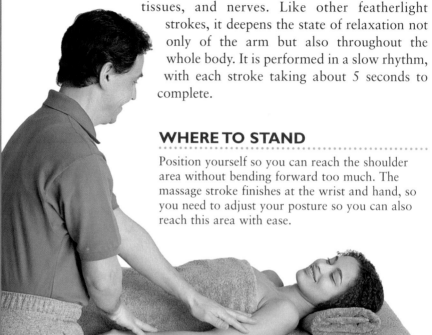

4

THE MASSAGE

With your fingers spread, place one hand on the shoulder, and the other farther down the arm. Using only the fingers of your upper hand, stroke very lightly all the way down the arm.

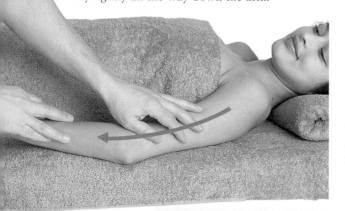

2 As the upper hand reaches the elbow, start featherlight stroking from the shoulder with your other hand. Continue each stroke as far as the hand. Repeat the alternating strokes a few times.

Head and Shoulders

5

HEAD AND SHOULDERS

Massage is not always applied to the whole body. It is equally effective and relaxing when carried out on a single region, such as the head and shoulders. This area is particularly affected by anxiety and stress. The muscles of the shoulders, which may already be rigid from bad postural habits, can tighten even more in response to stress. This situation often leads to the common ailment of tension headache. Stress can also cause the muscles of the scalp and face to tighten. By easing the muscle tightness in these areas, the soothing massage strokes can also relieve nervous strains and tension headaches. Massage along the line of the cheekbone also helps to drain the sinuses.

5

STARTING THE MASSAGE

The massage routine begins with this gentle stroke along the shoulders and up the sides of the neck. The movement relaxes the muscles and warms up the tissues, both of which are necessary before deeper massage can be applied.

PREPARING A PERSON FOR MASSAGE

For massage to the back of the shoulders and neck, the following posture should be adopted, unless otherwise specified.
- The person being massaged should lie face down.
- Support the forehead with a rolled-up towel. Alternatively, the person can support his head on his hands, or turn the head to one side, without any support.
- Place a folded towel or flat cushion under the abdomen and feet.
- Cover the rest of the body with a towel.

WHERE TO STAND

Position yourself at the head of the massage couch. To avoid too much bending forward, you may want to lower your body by spacing your feet apart and bending your knees slightly. Aim to keep your back straight.

THE MASSAGE

Place one hand on each shoulder, with your fingers on top and your thumbs on the underside, both pointing toward the feet. Your fingers should also be angled slightly toward the spine of the person you are massaging.

5

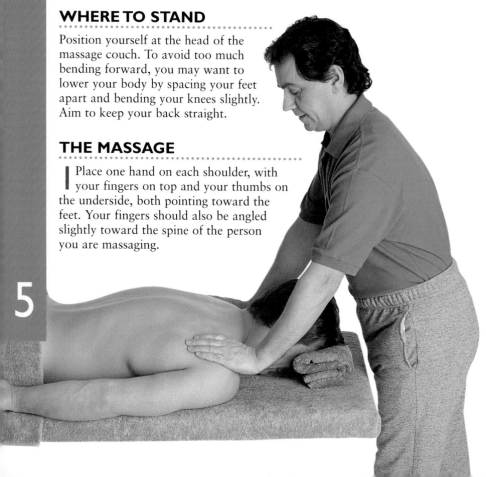

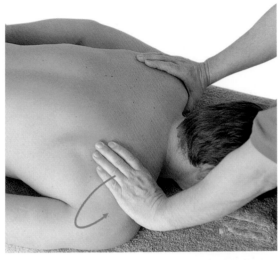

2 Without using any pressure, massage outward along each shoulder, keeping your fingers and thumbs at the same angle as in step 1. Continue the stroke as far as the upper arm.

3 As you reach the upper arm, reverse the position of your hands so the thumbs are on top and the fingers on the underside of the shoulders. The fingers need to curve slightly around the contours of the shoulder.

4 Slide the hands toward the neck. Do not apply pressure.

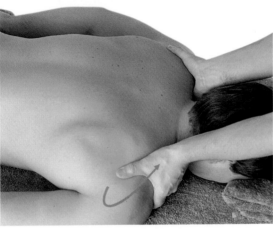

5 When you reach the neck, flatten your fingers and close the thumb to the hand. Continue the stroke along the sides of the neck and toward the head.

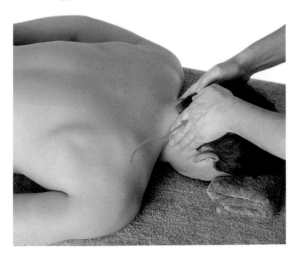

6 Remove your hands when you reach the base of the head. Position them on the shoulders in their start position and repeat the movement.

5

SHOULDERS: *Deep Stroke*

Tension is common in the muscles along the top of the shoulder, and massage to this area is therefore of great benefit in loosening and stretching the muscle fibers. As the shoulders respond particularly well to massage, there is very little risk of overdoing the treatment.

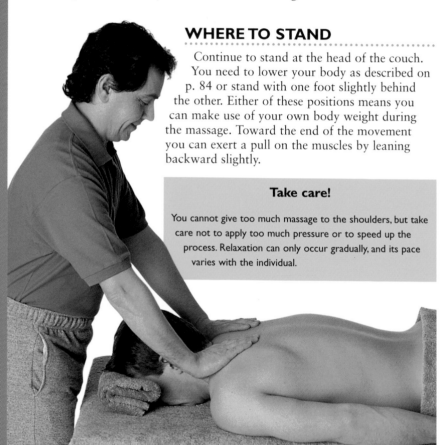

WHERE TO STAND

Continue to stand at the head of the couch. You need to lower your body as described on p. 84 or stand with one foot slightly behind the other. Either of these positions means you can make use of your own body weight during the massage. Toward the end of the movement you can exert a pull on the muscles by leaning backward slightly.

Take care!

You cannot give too much massage to the shoulders, but take care not to apply too much pressure or to speed up the process. Relaxation can only occur gradually, and its pace varies with the individual.

5

CAUSES OF TENSION IN THE SHOULDER

People in a sedentary job such as clerks or computer operators often suffer from stiff shoulders that feel tender to the touch. While massage can help, it is important to make sure your chair is at the correct height for the desk and the computer screen so you naturally sit up straight. The computer monitor should be at eye level and straight in front, not forcing you to twist to the side or look up or down. Those whose job necessitates standing in one spot for most of the day should also check that their posture is not the cause of tense shoulder muscles.

THE MASSAGE

1 Place your hands on the shoulders, one on each side. Position your hands so the fingers are on the upper side and the thumbs underneath. Have both fingers and thumbs pointing toward the feet of the person you are massaging.

2 Push the palms of your hands well into the muscles.

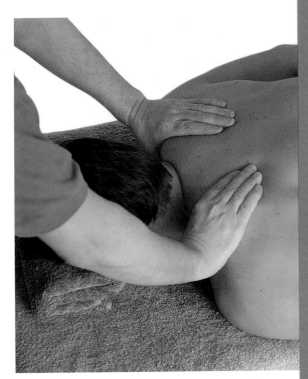

3 Squeeze the muscles between the fingers and thumb of each hand. Maintain this pressure as you slide your hands up toward you, stretching the muscles. Avoid pinching the skin.

4 Release your grip and repeat the movement.

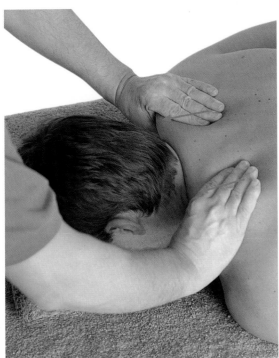

ALTERNATIVE

Instead of lying with his head straight, the person you are massaging may prefer to turn it to one side, without any support.

5

THE NECK: *Medium Stroke*

The muscles at the back of the neck help to stabilize the neck and act as supports for the head. They are also the main muscles that move the head and lift up the shoulders. Massage benefits these muscles by improving their circulation and promoting relaxation.

WHERE TO STAND

Shift your position so you are now standing at the side of the massage couch, close to the head of the person you are massaging. The same massage movement can also be carried out with the person seated (see box opposite).

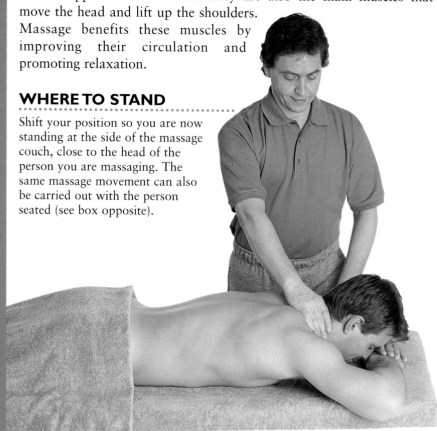

5

Warning!

Take extra care if the person receiving the massage suffers from any bone disorder such as arthritis. If this or any other condition is severe or painful the massage may have to be omitted to this area.

ALTERNATIVE

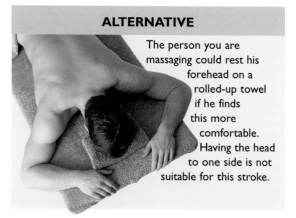

The person you are massaging could rest his forehead on a rolled-up towel if he finds this more comfortable. Having the head to one side is not suitable for this stroke.

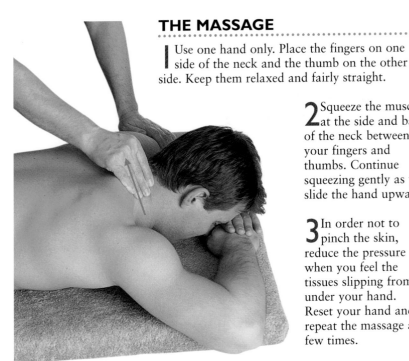

THE MASSAGE

1 Use one hand only. Place the fingers on one side of the neck and the thumb on the other side. Keep them relaxed and fairly straight.

2 Squeeze the muscles at the side and back of the neck between your fingers and thumbs. Continue squeezing gently as you slide the hand upward.

3 In order not to pinch the skin, reduce the pressure when you feel the tissues slipping from under your hand. Reset your hand and repeat the massage a few times.

SEATED POSITION

If the person you are massaging finds it uncomfortable to lie face down for this movement, or if there are no facilities to do so, he can sit instead. It is preferable for the person you are massaging to sit on a chair, rather than a stool, since a chair gives more support to the back and lessens any tendency to round the shoulders. Make sure the chair is at a comfortable height for you: you should not have to lean forward to massage effectively. Stand behind but slightly to one side of the person you are massaging, so that you keep your wrist straight. Keep your weight evenly distributed on both feet.

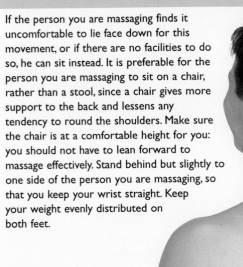

5

SHOULDERS: *Deep Stroke*

This massage is easy to carry out when the person you are massaging is sitting down. It is an ideal massage to give when time is limited or when there are no facilities for lying down. The stroke can therefore be carried out not only at home but almost anywhere. In addition to being very easy to perform, it is an extremely relaxing stroke, which can quickly release tension and pain in the shoulders. For these reasons it is a favorite massage with many people.

WHERE TO STAND

The person being massaged should sit on a chair rather than a stool, since this offers more support to the back and allows him to relax more readily. Stand behind the chair.

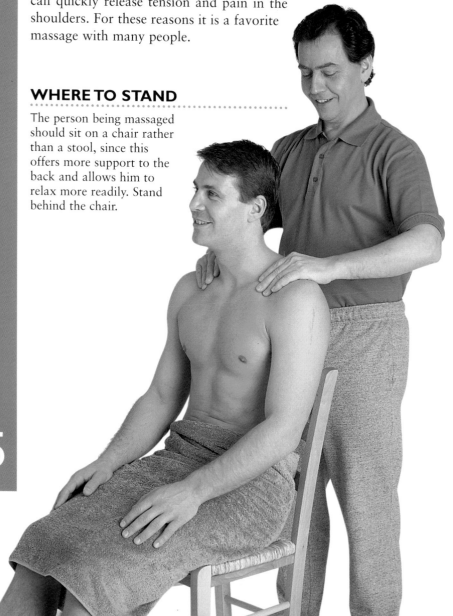

5

THE MASSAGE

1 Place one hand on each shoulder, with the fingers in front and the thumbs behind, between the spine and the shoulder blades. Keep the fingers fairly straight. Do not apply any weight on the shoulders.

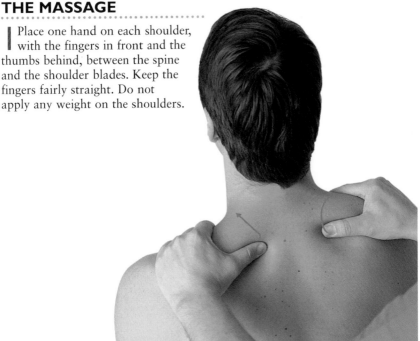

2 Squeeze the muscles upward between the fingers and thumbs. Keep the thumbs flat as you push the muscles upward. The fingers should be straight to avoid digging into the tissues at the front. Squeeze both shoulders simultaneously.

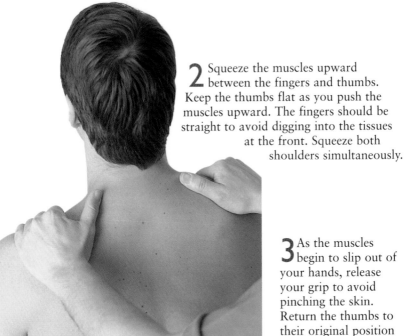

5

3 As the muscles begin to slip out of your hands, release your grip to avoid pinching the skin. Return the thumbs to their original position and repeat the stroke.

THE HEAD: *Light Stroke*

E ven though it is of great benefit, massage to the head and face is often underrated. Massage to the scalp, for example, is often neglected despite its ability to induce great relaxation. Tension, often registered in the forehead by signs of frowning, is readily reduced by the soothing massage strokes to this area. Gentle strokes along the cheekbone have a draining effect on the sinuses and help to unblock them.

WHERE TO STAND

The person receiving the massage sits on a chair with her arms hanging comfortably by her side or folded on her lap. Stand behind and close to the chair. Place a rolled-up towel or cushion behind the person's neck and ask her to tilt her head back slightly. If she finds this uncomfortable, remove the towel and let her rest her head against your abdomen or chest. Alternatively, she can keep it unsupported and straight.

THE MASSAGE

I No oil is necessary for these movements. Place the first and second fingers (or the second and third) in the center of the forehead. Position your fingers so they are more or less horizontal and close to each other. Apply a little pressure with your fingertips, and slowly slide your fingers out in a straight line toward the temples. Keep your fingers relaxed and flat on the skin surface. When you reach the temples, remove your hands. Repeat several times.

5

ALTERNATIVE

Depending on the size of your hands and of the forehead of the person you are massaging, you may prefer to use all four fingers of each hand instead of only two. Apply the same stroke, moving in a straight line from the center of the forehead out toward the temples.

2 To massage the scalp, spread your fingers and apply some pressure with the fingertips; do not use the thumbs for this massage. Maintain the pressure as you move the skin over the skull, using small circular movements. Work your way all around the scalp.

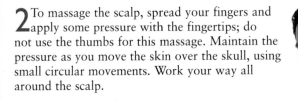

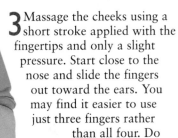

3 Massage the cheeks using a short stroke applied with the fingertips and only a slight pressure. Start close to the nose and slide the fingers out toward the ears. You may find it easier to use just three fingers rather than all four. Do not use your thumbs.

4 For jaw massage, place the tips of the first and second fingers on the bone just in front of the ear and slightly lower than the cheekline. To find this joint, ask the person you are massaging to open and close their mouth, and you will feel the bone moving under your fingers. The muscles that control chewing lie over this joint, and they are often tight from tension. Spend some time massaging this area. Use small circular movements or short strokes in the direction of the jawline.

5

SHOULDERS: *Light Stroke*

This light massage promotes relaxation and complements the facial routine described on pages 92–93. It can be applied before or after the massage to the face. The massage is easily adapted for a person sitting down, and carried out with other strokes for the shoulders.

WHERE TO STAND

Stand a slight distance away from the head end of the massage couch so you can comfortably place one hand on each shoulder. You may also want to lower your body by spacing your feet apart and bending your knees slightly. The person you are massaging lies on his back with his hands by his sides. Place a folded towel or cushion behind his head, and cover his legs with a towel.

THE MASSAGE

Place your hands on the outer borders of the shoulders, one hand on each side. Cup each hand and keep your thumb close to the palm. Massage around the shoulder and toward the neck.

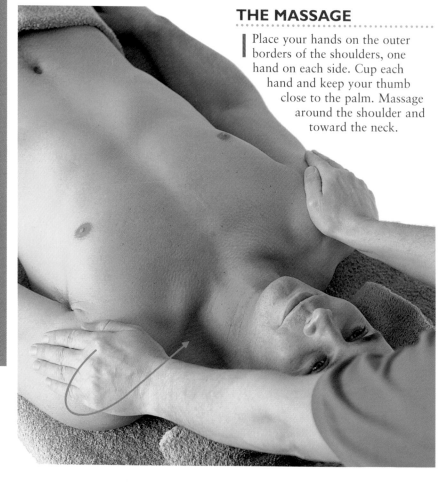

5

2 As you begin to massage along the top of the shoulders, keep your thumbs on the front and the fingers on the back. Let your hands follow the contours of the body as you massage in toward the neck. Use very little pressure and keep a slow rhythm.

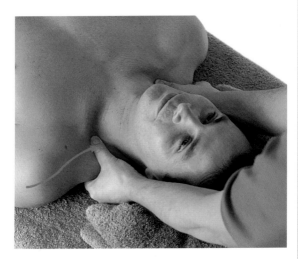

3 As you approach the neck, close the thumbs up to the palms again. Continue the massage into the neck and toward the head, sliding your fingers along the back of the neck. Trail your thumbs along the sides of the neck, without applying any pressure.

4 When you reach the base of the head, remove your hands. Repeat the stroke several times.

ALTERNATIVE POSITION

When the person is sitting, the light stroking massage is carried out from the shoulders toward the head (it can also be carried out in the opposite direction, if you prefer). Your hands should be curved slightly over the shoulders, and each thumb should be close to the palm. Use very little pressure on the shoulder and even less on the neck. Repeat the stroke several times.

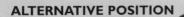

5

HEAD AND FACE MASSAGE

Massage of the face and head is an extremely pleasant way of ending the whole body massage routine and invariably deepens the level of relaxation gained earlier. It can also be given at the beginning of a whole routine, or on its own. If massage oil is used on the face, it should be applied sparingly.

WHERE TO STAND

Massage to the face is carried out with the person you are massaging lying down and with you standing at the head of the massage couch. Adjust your position so your hands remain relaxed as you place them on the person's face and apply the massage strokes. You may also find it easier to administer some of these movements sitting on a high stool or chair.

THE MASSAGE

1 Place the fingers of each hand in the middle of the forehead, pointing downward. Slide the fingers out across the forehead, moving toward the temples. When you reach the temple, remove your fingers or slide them lightly back to the middle, and repeat the stroke several times.

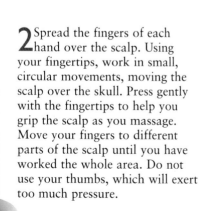

5

2 Spread the fingers of each hand over the scalp. Using your fingertips, work in small, circular movements, moving the scalp over the skull. Press gently with the fingertips to help you grip the scalp as you massage. Move your fingers to different parts of the scalp until you have worked the whole area. Do not use your thumbs, which will exert too much pressure.

3 Place your index finger and thumb on the bony ridge of the eye socket, with the thumb above and the finger below. Gently pinch the tissues over the bony ridge. Release your grip and repeat the squeezing movement once or twice. Repeat along the whole length of the bony ridge.

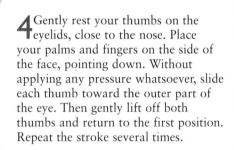

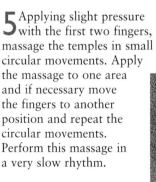

4 Gently rest your thumbs on the eyelids, close to the nose. Place your palms and fingers on the side of the face, pointing down. Without applying any pressure whatsoever, slide each thumb toward the outer part of the eye. Then gently lift off both thumbs and return to the first position. Repeat the stroke several times.

5 Applying slight pressure with the first two fingers, massage the temples in small circular movements. Apply the massage to one area and if necessary move the fingers to another position and repeat the circular movements. Perform this massage in a very slow rhythm.

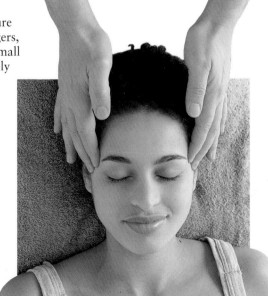

5

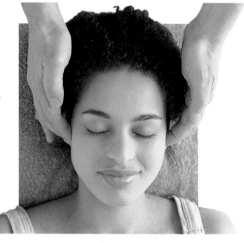

6 Position three or four fingers on each side of the face, close to the nose. Curve them so the tips fit just below the cheekbone. Using gentle pressure, slide the fingers along the cheekbone toward the ear. Just before you reach the ear, ease the pressure, and remove your hands. Repeat a few times.

7 Locate the jaw joint by placing your fingers on the prominent bone in this area and asking the person to open and close her mouth; you should feel the joint moving under your fingers. Applying a little pressure with the tips of your first two fingers, work in a series of small circular movements or in straight lines over the area, from ear level toward the lower jaw.

5

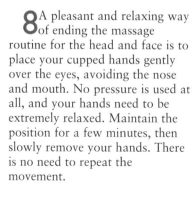

8 A pleasant and relaxing way of ending the massage routine for the head and face is to place your cupped hands gently over the eyes, avoiding the nose and mouth. No pressure is used at all, and your hands need to be extremely relaxed. Maintain the position for a few minutes, then slowly remove your hands. There is no need to repeat the movement.

Self Massage

6

ACUPRESSURE POINTS

At the middle point between your eye sockets is an acupressure "energy point," which is used to relieve mental tension and anxiety.

Place the tip of the index finger of each hand on either side of your nose, at the junction between the nose and the eye socket. Hold your fingertips in this position for a few seconds and press up toward your forehead.

Release the pressure, rest for a few seconds, and repeat. You should be able to feel tension ebbing.

MUSCLES OF THE JAW

The jaw muscles are located just in front of the ear and slightly down from the cheekbone. You can feel them over the bone as the jaw moves up and down. Massage helps to reduce the tension that often builds up in these muscles. Use your first and second, or second and third fingers, to massage this area. Apply gentle pressure with the fingertips and work in small, circular movements.

SCALP

Massage to the scalp completes this relaxing routine to the face and head. Spread your fingers and place them on your head, starting either on the top or the sides. Do not use your thumbs. Apply pressure with your fingertips and massage your scalp using small circular movements. Continue the movement for a few seconds before moving to another section, until you have massaged your whole scalp.

6

BACK OF NECK AND HEAD

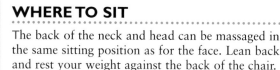

Muscles arising from the upper back and shoulders run along the back of the neck and attach to the base of the skull. These muscles stabilize and move the head. As they are also involved in the movements of the shoulders, they are often overused and tight. Massage to this area is very relaxing and particularly useful for relieving tension headache.

WHERE TO SIT

The back of the neck and head can be massaged in the same sitting position as for the face. Lean back and rest your weight against the back of the chair.

THE MASSAGE

1 Place your hands at the back of your neck, one on each side. Make contact with the fingers of each hand, keeping them horizontal. Position them where they can cover the muscles on the sides and the back of your neck. Take your time and massage the whole area. Press into the tissues as you massage, using small circular movements.

2 Place your fingertips just below the bony ridge at the base of your head: this bony ridge is where all the muscles attach to the bone, making it a particularly receptive area for massage. Arrange your fingers at a vertical angle, pointing toward the top of your head. Press with your fingertips as you massage the tissues and bone with the same circular movements as before.

6

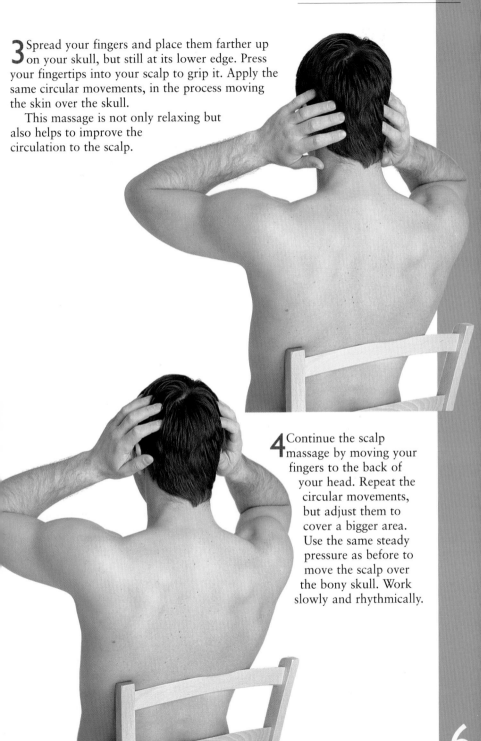

3 Spread your fingers and place them farther up on your skull, but still at its lower edge. Press your fingertips into your scalp to grip it. Apply the same circular movements, in the process moving the skin over the skull.

This massage is not only relaxing but also helps to improve the circulation to the scalp.

4 Continue the scalp massage by moving your fingers to the back of your head. Repeat the circular movements, but adjust them to cover a bigger area. Use the same steady pressure as before to move the scalp over the bony skull. Work slowly and rhythmically.

6

THE SHOULDERS

A nxiety, nervous strain, bad posture, and overuse can make the shoulder muscles tight and tense. This self massage is easy to carry out, and effective in encouraging the muscles to relax. The movement can be performed as a massage on its own: the neck and head do not need to be included. Another advantage of this stroke is that it can be done without removing any clothing.

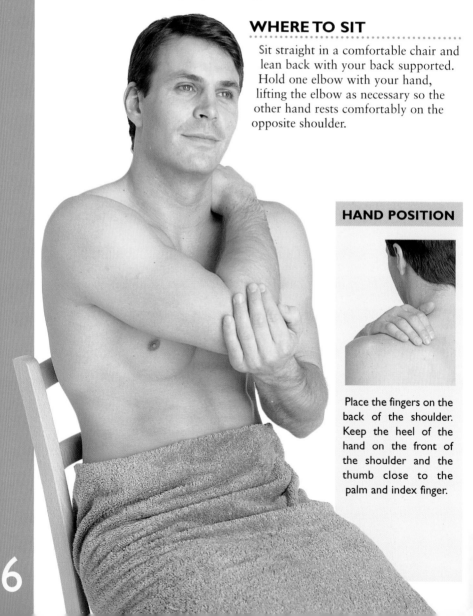

WHERE TO SIT

Sit straight in a comfortable chair and lean back with your back supported. Hold one elbow with your hand, lifting the elbow as necessary so the other hand rests comfortably on the opposite shoulder.

HAND POSITION

Place the fingers on the back of the shoulder. Keep the heel of the hand on the front of the shoulder and the thumb close to the palm and index finger.

6

THE MASSAGE

1 Squeeze your shoulder muscles with your fingers and the heel of your hand. Apply the pressure gradually, and adjust it to suit the tension in the muscles. Arrange the position of your hand so the muscle tissue is compressed without too much force being applied on the front of your shoulder or on the collarbone. Hold the grip for a few seconds.

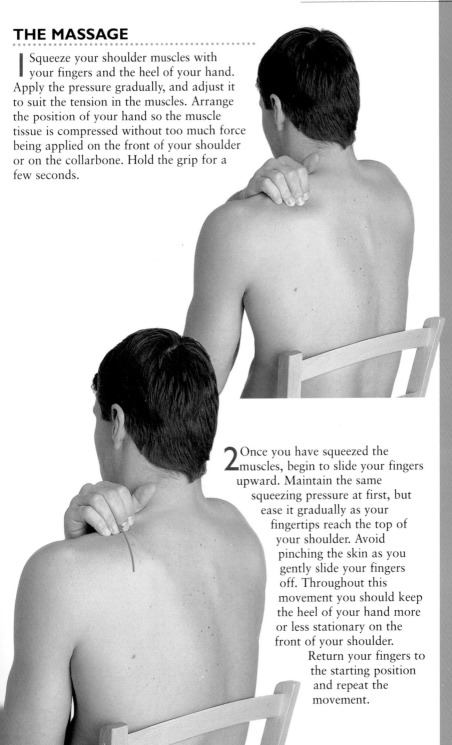

2 Once you have squeezed the muscles, begin to slide your fingers upward. Maintain the same squeezing pressure at first, but ease it gradually as your fingertips reach the top of your shoulder. Avoid pinching the skin as you gently slide your fingers off. Throughout this movement you should keep the heel of your hand more or less stationary on the front of your shoulder.

Return your fingers to the starting position and repeat the movement.

6

THE HANDS

In addition to being relaxing, massage to the hands helps to nourish the muscles and tissues by improving their circulation. It also loosens the joints and the small muscles of the palm and fingers.

Such remedial treatments can be of great help in cases of arthritis and rheumatism. They go some way to relieving pain, especially if used in conjunction with the appropriate creams or oils. To increase the benefit of this massage, you may want to soak your hands in warm water for a few minutes beforehand.

Reflex zones or points are located over the front and back of the hand and fingers. These reflex points relate to energy channels within the body, in a similar manner to those reflex points on the feet. Massage to the hand can therefore be seen as having a balancing effect on the body's energies.

WHERE TO SIT

Sit somewhere comfortable, for example, on a chair, couch, or bed. Rest your hands on your lap or on a table in front of you. Use a pillow or folded towel to support your hands, unless you prefer to hold them up closer to you.

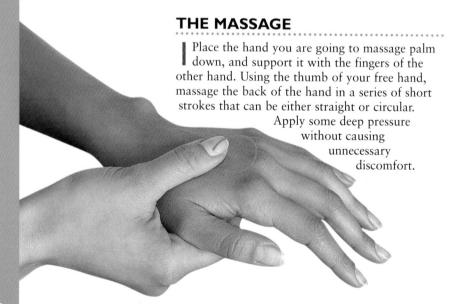

THE MASSAGE

Place the hand you are going to massage palm down, and support it with the fingers of the other hand. Using the thumb of your free hand, massage the back of the hand in a series of short strokes that can be either straight or circular. Apply some deep pressure without causing unnecessary discomfort.

6

2 Turn your hand over so you can massage the palm with your thumb, using small circular movements. There are more muscles here than on the back of the hand, so you can apply slightly deeper pressure. You can also continue the strokes to include the fingers.

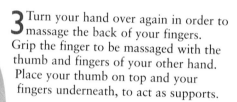

3 Turn your hand over again in order to massage the back of your fingers. Grip the finger to be massaged with the thumb and fingers of your other hand. Place your thumb on top and your fingers underneath, to act as supports.

4 Applying some pressure, slide your thumb back and forth on your finger. Do this by bending your thumb at the middle joint, then straightening it again. Repeat the back and forth stroke a few more times and along the whole length of your finger. Then apply the same massage to all your other fingers. You can also massage the palm side of your fingers like this by turning your hand palm up.

6

THE FOREARM

The two layers of muscles on the front and the back of the forearm are involved in gripping with the hand and bending the wrist backward and forward. They are therefore used in all physical work and sports activity. As a result, they can tighten because of fatigue and will nearly always benefit from some massage which helps to decongest them and loosen them up.

OUTER FOREARM: THUMB PRESSURE

1 Sit comfortably on a chair or stool. Place your thumb on the back of your forearm. Keep your thumb flat against the skin and wrap your fingers around your forearm.

2 Press into the muscles with your thumb to apply some pressure. At the same time squeeze your forearm with your fingers as a counterforce. Maintain the pressure and slide your thumb in a circular direction, then ease the pressure temporarily. Press the thumb into the muscles again and repeat the circular movement.

3 Move your hand to another part of your forearm and repeat. Continue over the whole forearm. If your muscles are tight or well developed, increase the pressure with your thumb by bending it slightly. Hold this position and slide it in a circular direction.

OUTER FOREARM: FINGER PRESSURE

1 The back of your forearm can also be massaged using your fingertips instead of your thumb. Hold your forearm with your other hand, placing the fingers on the back of the forearm and the thumb on the front.

2 Keep your fingers close to each other, and apply pressure with the fingertips. Move your fingers back and forth over the muscles. Adjust the pressure by bending your fingers to increase it, and flattening them to lessen it. Move your hand to different parts of your forearm and repeat the same stroke.

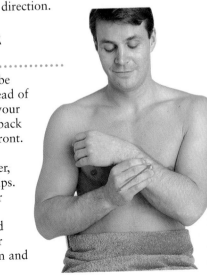

6

TENDONS

The tendons of the forearm muscles are located around the elbow. They attach to the elbow and can be felt to the front of the elbow joint. Their blood supply is not as rich as that of muscles. Massage can therefore be of benefit to these tendons by increasing their circulation. To massage your tendons, use your thumb in small circular movements, or in a back and forth movement. Alternatively, you can use your fingertips to apply the stroke. Increase the pressure gradually and without causing undue discomfort.

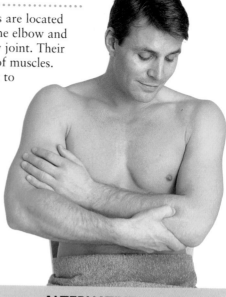

ALTERNATIVE

To massage your forearm you may prefer to rest it on your lap instead of holding it up. Apply pressure with your thumb, keeping it flat on the muscles. Either use small circular movements or slide your thumb back and forth.

INNER FOREARM

1 To massage the front of your forearm, turn it around. Place your thumb on the front of your forearm and the fingers on the back. Squeeze your forearm with your thumb and fingers. Maintain the squeeze as you massage with the thumb.

2 Massage by sliding your thumb in a circular direction. When you have completed one circle, momentarily ease off the pressure. Then press your thumb into the tissues again and repeat the same circular massage. Continue over the whole forearm.

6

THE FOOT

Each foot is arched and has over 20 bones – the feet are complex structures that have to support the weight of the entire body and act as shock absorbers. They can easily get tired from being cramped inside shoes, from overuse, or even from walking. Fluid accumulation can be another problem that often results from long periods of standing. Massaging your feet helps to decongest them and improves their circulation. It also has an invigorating effect, not only on the feet but on the whole body. This occurs because it stimulates tiny reflex zones that are located all over each foot and which relate to organs or body regions.

WHERE TO SIT

Sit on a chair or stool. This needs to be of a height which enables you to rest one foot on your opposite thigh. You could also sit on the floor. Arrange your sitting position so you can reach the upper part of your foot comfortably and without causing any strain on your back.

THE MASSAGE: USING BOTH THUMBS

Hold your foot with both hands, placing the thumbs on the sole and keeping them flat on the skin surface. Massage in a circular direction with the right thumb, applying some pressure. Then ease the pressure and repeat the stroke with your left thumb. Continue to alternate the thumb strokes as you massage all over your sole. If you come across a spot that is tender, spend some extra time on it until the sensitivity reduces. If it is too painful, move to another area.

6

USING ONE THUMB

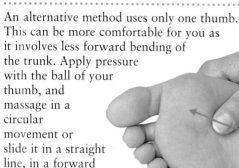

An alternative method uses only one thumb. This can be more comfortable for you as it involves less forward bending of the trunk. Apply pressure with the ball of your thumb, and massage in a circular movement or slide it in a straight line, in a forward direction.

UPPER PART OF FOOT

A similar thumb action can be applied on the upper part of your foot. Move your thumb in circular movements or in short straight lines, in a forward direction. Use one or both thumbs to massage this area. For this massage, you may prefer to place your foot on a stool in front of you instead of resting it on your lap.

FOOT PROBLEMS

- The feet can easily become tired from being cramped inside shoes for long periods. Do not wear shoes that are too small or do not fit properly.
- Fluid accumulation, which results from a lot of walking or standing, also causes tired feet.
- Some conditions affecting the whole body system or certain organs such as the kidney or heart can cause fluid to accumulate in the legs and feet.
- Poor foot mechanics, such as fallen arches, may cause pain in the feet, and elsewhere.

Warning!

If massage of any spot is painful, stop and move to another area. Some parts of your foot will probably be more sensitive than others, but the tenderness should not reach the level of unpleasant pain.

6

INDEX

Note: Words in **bold** represent major text entries

ACKNOWLEDGMENTS

The author and publishers wish to acknowledge the invaluable contribution made to this book by Laura Wickenden, who took all the photographs.

The author and publishers would also like to thank the models Christiane and Patrick Jones, and stylist Tanya Volhard.

Mario-Paul Cassar can be contacted at:
Massage and Bodywork Institute, 93 Parkhurst Road, Horley, Surrey RH6 8EX, England.